A Waist Is a Terrible
Thing to Mind

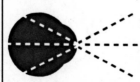

This Large Print Book carries the
Seal of Approval of N.A.V.H.

A WAIST IS A TERRIBLE THING TO MIND

LOVING YOUR BODY, ACCEPTING YOURSELF, AND LIVING WITHOUT REGRET

KAREN SCALF LINAMEN

CHRISTIAN LARGE PRINT

A part of Gale, Cengage Learning

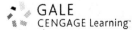
GALE
CENGAGE Learning

Detroit • New York • San Francisco • New Haven, Conn • Waterville, Maine • London

GALE
CENGAGE Learning

Thorndike Press, a part of Gale, Cengage Learning.

Christian Large Print Originals.
The text of this Large Print edition is unabridged.
Other aspects of the book may vary from the original edition.
Set in 16 pt. Plantin.

LIBRARY OF CONGRESS CATALOGING-IN-PUBLICATION DATA

Linamen, Karen Scalf, 1960–
   A waist is a terrible thing to mind : loving your body, accepting yourself, and living without regret / By Karen Scalf Linamen. — Large print ed.
       p. cm. — (Christian Large Print originals)
   Includes bibliographical references.
   ISBN-13: 978-1-59415-326-6 (softcover)
   ISBN-10: 1-59415-326-4 (softcover)
   1. Human body—Religious aspects—Christianity. 2. Health—Religious aspects—Christianity. 3. Beauty, Personal—Religious aspects—Christianity. 4. Christian women—Religious life. 5. Large type books. I. Title. II. Series.
   BT741.3.L56 2010b
   261.5'61—dc22   2010008563

Published in 2010 by arrangement with WaterBrook Press, an imprint of the Crown Publishing Group, a division of Random House, Inc.

Printed in the United States of America
   1 2 3 4 5   14 13 12 11 10
ED155

*This book is dedicated to you,
yes, you, the beautiful woman
reading this page.*

*My hope is that this book would
become for you — if not a key —
at least a compass
and that your journey would prove rich
and transforming in every way.*

CONTENTS

ACKNOWLEDGMENTS

A book is crafted by many hands and hearts, and I wish I had the space to list the names of everyone who has contributed to this work. I don't, of course, but here's the short list.

I simply must thank all the irritating and/or clueless folks in my life who have, wittingly and unwittingly, driven me to cookies. And ice cream. And especially chocolate. I'm not saying that seeking solace via chocolate is a good thing or even something one should try on a regular basis. But I can say that without my own struggles to make peace with my body and my emotions, this book could never have been written. At least not by me.

The people who have contributed to this project in a much more enjoyable fashion include my agent, Steve Laube, and Ron Lee, senior editor at WaterBrook Multnomah. Both of these men have proven themselves mentors, friends, and handholders extraordinaire. Kudos also to WaterBrook Multnomah production editor Laura Wright for her talents (and patience!) and to publicity manager Melissa "Pirate Wench" Sturgis and her amazing team of Elizabeth Johnson, Lynette Kittle, and Allison O'Hara. Thanks also to Joe Ramirez, a personal trainer who makes house calls, for rescuing me out of my carb coma and forcing me to "work it" in the discomfort of my own living room.

Finally, very special thanks to all the transparent and beautiful women who allowed me the profound privilege of getting to know them and sharing their stories in the pages of this book. Exploring their stories — and my own — has been the stuff of transformation in my own life, and for that I am eternally grateful.

1
What's a Nice Girl Like Me Doing in a Size Like This?

MAKING PEACE WITH YO-YO DIETING

Okay, fine. I admit it. I'm the girl of a thousand diets. I've tried them all: Atkins, Grapefruit, Egg, Weight Watchers, Nutrisystem, Diet Center. On and on, to *ad diet nauseum.*

Actually, the diet with which I've had the most success is the Yo-Yo Diet, also known as the Déjà Moo Diet, the diet I turn to whenever I get the feeling that I have — once again — put on weight and feel like a cow. I wish I could tell you that going on all these diets has made me svelte. Actually they have, if *svelte* stands for Still Voraciously Eating Lotsa Treats Enthusiastically.

Unfortunately, many of my friends share the same problem. Maybe they're not bouncing up and down the scale on yo-yo diets like I am, but almost every woman I know has something she would love to change about her body, her shape, or the way she looks.

Knowing this about other people brings a bit of relief. Not that I *want* my friends to suffer. (In fact, I wouldn't wish this problem on anyone, not even the woman who whipped her car in front of mine and stole the first-row parking space I was about to claim in the Krispy Kreme parking lot.) But knowing that other women (and men) struggle to change their bodies — or, at the very least, struggle to change how they feel about their bodies — makes me feel a little less . . . well . . . alone.

Apparently we're all in this together. Even celebrities have this problem, which always amazes the rest of us because most celebrities have the money to hire personal chefs and personal trainers and personal fashion consultants, not to mention their own fleet of personal air-brush artists. I wouldn't be surprised if the wealthiest stars even hire personal binge doubles who wear the pounds in the relationship. Here's how it works: a movie star pigs out for a weekend and her binge double gains seven pounds. (If Dorian Gray had been raking in a movie-star salary, he would have gone this route instead of the more budget-friendly oil on canvas.)

Yet, even with *all* these resources, many Hollywood hotties do the yo-yo thing too:

fat, thin, fat, thin, fat, thin. And I understand their pain. It can unnerve a girl, never knowing what size she's going to be tomorrow morning. Consider Alice, for example. Within minutes of arriving in Wonderland, she took one measly bite of cake and blew up three times her normal size. It made her so upset that she cried a literal river of tears. (I can *so* relate!) But if there was all this drama over a single bite of cake, imagine how huge and hysterical Alice would get if, like me, she were in the habit of consuming an entire party-size box of Twinkies in a single sitting.

I don't know about you, but as for me and Alice, there's not much we'd love more than getting our bodies to a size that feels healthy and good . . . and staying there. What about you?

- Does your closet contain more sizes than your local department store?
- Do you change diets more often than you change the cardboard empties in your toilet-paper dispenser?
- Have you been up and down the scale more often than a beginning piano student?
- Do you long for a committed, long-term relationship with your skinny

15

jeans instead of all these short-lived flings?

- How many different diets have *you* tried? In fact, if you added up all the pounds you've lost over and over again, would you make the cover of *The Weekly World News*? Would the headline read something like this: "Woman loses 6,811 pounds and lives to tell the story"? Don't feel bad. They ran the same story on me last month.

EISOPTROPHOBICS SHOULD NEVER APPLY THEIR OWN EYELINER

I can put on weight for months, all the while pretending not to notice. As you can imagine, this requires a carefully calibrated system of justification and excusification, not to mention an active avoidance of any reality-based information that might undermine my denial. This is why, if I have a doctor's appointment and the nurse needs to update my chart, sometimes I stand on the scale with my eyes closed, humming "The Star Spangled Banner." If she insists on knowing my weight, that's her business. All I know is that I don't have a burning need to see the numbers — or hear her announce the numbers. And I certainly don't want to hear her gasp and turn toward the nurses' station while she points at me: "Hey girls! Come take a look at this! Did anyone know the digits on this scale went this high?"

Of course, if I really wanted to stay ignorant of the shape of my body, I could develop eisoptrophobia, which is a fear of mirrors. Except what if I were afraid of mirrors and then lost fifty pounds and wanted to admire my new shape? Or what if I ever wanted to go to counseling and my therapist asked me to take a good look at myself and do some personal reflection?

Apparently I do not suffer from eisoptrophobia. I say this because last year I looked in the mirror and realized I was the heaviest I'd been in a long time. In fact, at 227 pounds, it dawned on me that I'd broken one of the first commandments of weight management, which is: "Thou shalt not weigh more than thy refrigerator." (You think I'm joking? My make and model of fridge weighs 187 pounds. I looked it up.)

I don't know why my weight came as a surprise to me. After all, I'd not only been feeling fat and tired, but sad and hopeless too. You see, every time I lose weight, I feel great about my body and my life, while every time I gain it back, I feel angst and shame. And since my angst and shame had skyrocketed, it shouldn't have come as a surprise that the numbers on my scale had done the same thing.

So I did what I always do when this happens, I started a new diet. At the time, this always seems like a good idea. And it probably would be a good idea if dieting didn't require the mastery of a particular substance that may seem simple, but in reality is about as simple as brain surgery or programming the TiVo.

That substance, of course, is food.

SO MANY DIETS, SO LITTLE FOCUS

I don't know what your relationship with food is like, but to me, food always feels really complicated.

I know it's supposed to be simple. Something to do with fueling our bodies. I hear it's supposed to work like this: feel hungry, eat nutrients, get energy, move around, feel hungry again, eat more nutrients. In fact, it's kind of like what we do with our cars: fill up and drive. Fill up and drive. Fill up and drive. Food is supposed to work like that, except it tastes better than gas and doesn't make us complain about the price at the pumps.

To me, food has always seemed more

complex than that. Take breakfast, for example. The remarkably simple question "Gee, what should I have for breakfast?" can turn into the kind of conundrum that would reduce Ernö Rubik to tears. Indeed, last year when I decided to start a new diet, I headed into the kitchen for breakfast, opened the fridge, and — true to form — felt a surge of panic. Here is a random sampling of the thoughts that went ping-ponging around my brain as I studied the contents of my General Electric:

Hmm . . . what kind of diet should I start? Maybe a low-carb diet? If so, for breakfast I could eat a three-cheese omelet and a half pound of bacon.

Then again, I could always make it a low-glycemic-index day and start off with oatmeal and a piece of rye toast.

Or maybe I should nix food altogether and stick with diet drinks all day.

Come to think of it, that egg diet worked well for me once, although nine hard-boiled eggs in one day can get a little tedious.

Of course, I could always grab one of the Nutrisystem breakfasts I bought off that woman on Craigslist.

No, wait! I still have some of that grasslike substance from last year's colon-cleanse program. All I have to do is mix it with apple juice to create a nutrient- and fiber-rich cocktail that tastes like it was scraped off the bottom of my lawnmower.

With these thoughts swimming around in my brain like Goldfish crackers, it's no wonder I felt confused and decided to do the only thing that made any sense at the moment: I fasted.

When you can't figure out what to eat, don't eat anything. I do this a lot. It works beautifully for me until about two in the afternoon, when I become so famished I scarf down a pound of bacon, four Nutrisystems, a Tupperware storage container full of leftover mac and cheese, a couple of bowls of Rice Krispies, and half a pan of brownies eaten with a spoon that I dip repeatedly in peanut butter. Which explains why — whenever I decide to get control of my body and my life — it usually only takes about seven hours to feel fatter and more discouraged than ever.

But last year, as I stared into my refrigerator and pondered a new diet, something clicked. If I were going to kick this thing once and for all, I needed a new approach. Something I'd never tried before.

It's not like I don't already know how to lose weight, what with losing the same forty to sixty pounds over and over and over. But

I realized there were apparently some things I didn't know, because I'd been fighting the same battle again and again. I was not only exhausted from the fray, I was disillusioned with the chaos that characterized just about all my experiences with my body and with food.

And that's when I came to a life-changing conclusion: I didn't need to figure out how to lose forty pounds. What I really needed was to figure out how to make peace with my body once and for all.

THE ODDS AREN'T EXACTLY IN OUR FAVOR

The more I've thought about it, the more I've realized how unpeaceful this part of my life has been. In fact, I struggle with angst and confusion in a lot of areas as a result of how I manage food, manage my body, and manage my emotions about my body.

For example, just when I get my willpower working for me and I'm eating healthier meals, I get stressed, and my taste buds start screaming for junk food. Shortly after I get my taste buds under control, my schedule gets crowded, and I stop going to the gym. By the time my schedule clears up, I've gotten discouraged over some relationship in my life, and I've turned to the mac and cheese. Just about the time I'm over that little setback, summer has arrived, and the thought of donning short sleeves or a swimsuit is enough to send me into therapy.

And I'm not alone. Women everywhere agree: when it comes to managing our waistlines (or our emotions about our waistlines), the struggle can feel endless. Have you ever stopped to think about all the factors that work against us? Whether we're struggling to reshape our bodies or feel good about our bodies just as they are, you and I face opposition, temptation, or distraction in almost every area of our lives.

For starters, our cravings work against us, sending us foraging for Ding Dongs and Little Debbies.

Our busy schedules keep us from going to the gym and send us instead to the drive-through lane of the nearest fast-food restaurant.

Our society's obsession with just one shape (skinny) makes us feel fat even if we're not.

Entire industries conspire against us, enticing us with fatty foods and sumo-wrestler quantities, not to mention growth hormones that create plumper cattle but also make the people who eat them — pardon the pun — beefier as well.

Emotional wounds and relationship ghosts can work against us, too, prompting us to try to protect ourselves from future hurt by piling on the weight. (Somehow, we believe the extra weight keeps potential heartaches at bay.)

Our lifestyles work against us, keeping us comfortably inactive and sweat free. And I haven't even mentioned age and gravity!

Finally, you and I war against ourselves, giving in to deceptive thinking and self-defeating beliefs.

With all this stuff conspiring to make us fat or make us think we're fat, is it any wonder our efforts to feel good about our bodies seem to go largely unrewarded?

Making peace with our bodies doesn't mean achieving a magic number on the scale. It does mean having the energy we need to live the lives we desire. It means feeling confident about the way we look. It means getting our cravings, schedules, and beliefs working *for* us instead of against us. It means (gasp!) making love with the lights on and loving every minute of it.

So how do we begin?

GET A NEW BODITUDE

Questions for Personal Reflection or Group Discussion

• Do you like your body? Why or why not?

• Think about the other areas of your life that are affected by the way you feel about your body. (For example, your relationships with men, friendships with women, how confident you feel in your career, how active you are with your kids, how much stress you feel at the start of the day, how happy or content you are in general.)

• If you have tried (and failed) to get in better shape, what factors contributed to your lack of success?

• If you could find a way to be at peace with your body, how would it change your life?

2
WHO YOU GONNA CALL?
RUT BUSTERS!
MAKING PEACE WITH GETTING STARTED

It's not rocket science. If we keep doing the same things we've always done, we're going to keep getting the same results we've always gotten. Do we want new results? Then we've got to try some new approaches.

Which is why, last year, I decided to try something completely different. I decided to hire a personal trainer. But not just *any* personal trainer. I needed someone who could teach me how to do more than lift a dumbbell. I needed help figuring out all the things it takes to develop a healthy lifestyle once and for all.

I googled "health and weight loss resources" in my city. Before long, I'd landed on something promising. On the Web site www.joesbootcamp.com, Joe Ramirez introduced himself as an in-home personal trainer as well as a weight-loss and lifestyle consultant. I e-mailed him, and he called me that afternoon.

After hearing my story, Joe said he could help me. He sounded so confident I actually felt a surge of hope.

"Then let's do this," I said. "Let's do two or three sessions a week for one month. A month might seem like a drop in the bucket considering the massive whole-life overhaul I just told you I need, but it's what I can afford. I'm a starving artist — okay, a chubby starving artist, which I know seems like an oxymoron — but the point is, I can afford one month."

Joe said, "We'll figure something out. The important thing is to get started, then do what we need to do to get you where you want to be."

WHAT DOES IT TAKE TO CHANGE YOUR LIFE?

I wish you and I could talk as I'm writing this book. But since we can't, I don't know if you are longing to change your body, or change how you feel about your body, or both. But whether you want to lose, gain, tone, get healthier, feel sexier, have more energy — or simply learn to appreciate and cherish what you have — it's possible you picked up this book because you're having a hard time getting started all by yourself.

Except you're not all by yourself. Millions

of people are in the same boat as you, people who can't seem to get started by themselves. In fact, if you ask me, it's a very crowded boat. And since we're all not starting by ourselves together, maybe we can put our heads in the same place and figure out how to stop not-starting together and, instead, start starting together.

What does it take to stop milling about and start reclaiming our lives? How do we change our shapes, our lifestyles, or the way we think and feel about our bodies?

I called several women I know who have made peace with their bodies. I needed to know the answer to a single question: "What was the turning point for you? How did you get out of the rut you were in and make whatever changes you needed to make to feel comfortable in your own body?" I wish I could tell you that their answers all boiled down to a common strategy so that you and I would know exactly what to do. But, alas, their answers were as varied as the flavors in a bag of jelly beans.

I met Jessica at my gym. She was in her late twenties when she made the decision to reclaim her body and her health. She told me, "I visited my family one Christmas and got a real wake-up call. After watching my fifty-four-year-old mom using a walker because obesity and diabetes have trashed her body, I knew I needed to change my destiny. I was just forty pounds overweight and not a hundred and forty — but I knew if I didn't make a U-turn and make it stick, I would get there eventually."

My friend Kristen described a different kind of wake-up call: "When my daughter turned fifteen and started blossoming into a woman, I thought it would be a wonderful bonding time for us. But instead of bonding over makeup and girlie things, I got impatient and snappy. It dawned on me that I was jealous because she was coming into her femininity while I'd buried mine under dozens of pounds of fat. That did it. For me to shepherd my daughter wisely through this time in her life, I needed to be physically and emotionally fit so as not to scar her with my own baggage." Kristen took up yoga, got into counseling, and dropped forty-two pounds.

Jill's rut ended the day her husband of thirty-two years came to her and said, "I love you, but for twenty years I've been begging you to stop neglecting your body and our sex life. I can't do it one more day. I want us to have an open marriage. I'll be looking for a mistress."

Jill told me later, "Friends told me to show

him the door, but everything he'd said about how I'd treated my body and our sex life was true, and I wanted to save my marriage. It was an excruciating time for us, but I tried to stay focused on losing weight, awakening my sensual self, and rediscovering my husband. By the end of that year, I weighed fifty-five pounds less and we had rediscovered each other as lovers. We have renewed our commitment to each other and to meeting each other's needs, and our marriage has never been stronger. As for me, I'm fifty-seven years old, and I've never felt better about my body."

FIND A NEW PERSPECTIVE

For some women, making peace with their bodies doesn't involve changing dress sizes but changing their perspectives. Anne, for example, told me that making peace with her body began the day she hunted through magazines, looking for photos of "real" women of every age and shape. She pinned the pictures to her bulletin board and taped them to her fridge and mirrors.

Susan, a self-described "conservative, religious, thirty-five-year-old with a far-from-perfect body," says that visiting a nude beach and experiencing the sun and wind in places where, well . . . the sun typically doesn't shine, was the beginning of embracing a healthier and saner attitude toward her body.

Andrea wrote the following: "Yes, I have worn sexier undies and practiced positive affirmations, but the main reason I love and respect my curvy, size 18 body now is because I finally realized that a life of dieting and hating my body is not for me! And although I have taken many steps to get to where I now love and accept my curvy body, the transformation began when I realized that the negative critic that lived inside me was the voice of my father, and that the first step to making friends with my body was to stop thinking of myself as a victim, or as not good enough, pretty enough, or smart enough."

Danielle shared that her turning point involved deciding to wear clothes that were the right size for her body. She admitted that her closet contains at least a week's worth of office wear in every size from eight to eighteen. She says, "Looking frumpy, dumpy, or squeezing into ill-fitting clothes makes me feel awful. I look awful! I am in pain! But now my self-confidence has increased because I refuse to wear clothing that is baggy and shapeless just so I can hide my body. And my comfort and happiness increase because I never wear clothes that are so tight that I'm in pain, pinched, breathless, or sporting big red marks gouged into my skin at the end of the day. Wearing properly fitting clothes definitely helped me stop warring with my shape and my figure."

Mary discovered that writing poetry helped her come to terms with her body despite complications and limitations from polio and post-polio syndrome.

You'll read more about some of these women and their journeys in later chapters. For now, realize that making peace with our bodies is a story that each of us can write.

Calling Joe was an important plot twist for me, but what is your story going to be? Two months from now, or two years or even ten, when you look back at the incident or insight that got your attention and changed your life forever, what will it be? Has it already taken place? Could it be happening now? If not, how much longer are you willing to wait?

FAT CALIPERS . . . YIPPEE

I had my first in-home session with Joe on a Monday morning. Accompanied by his assistant, Jan, Joe arrived looking exactly like you'd expect a trainer to look — six foot tall and muscled — toting his laptop and a gym bag filled with mysterious doodads.

The first doodad to emerge was something that looked like a misshapen pair of tongs.

"Are we serving spaghetti?" I quipped.

"Nope. Measuring body fat."

I winced. "I preferred the spaghetti." As apparently I'd been doing for quite some time.

After pinching folds of flesh on my arms, belly, and thighs, Joe plugged in some numbers on his laptop and showed me the results. Turns out I was, like, 40 percent fat. Oh joy. Of course, healthy bodies need fat, but since the number should be around 22 percent, I knew we had some work to do.

"Ready for your first workout?" Joe asked. I nodded, and he reached back into his bag of tricks. I was expecting him to haul out dumbbells and barbells (and wondering how he'd carried the bag into the house so effortlessly), but instead he produced resistance bands, a medicine ball, and a couple of plastic disks that looked like Frisbees.

Over the next forty minutes — using just those three items — he turned my living room into a gym, replicating pretty much any move I can do on the expensive exercise machines. It was amazing. It was also foreboding.

"This is the easy workout?" I asked, gasping for air as I crouched, my palms on the carpet and feet on those Frisbee things, sliding my legs back and forth like some weird stationary insect.

Joe sniffed at the air. "Do I smell something burning? No, wait, that's you! You're doing great. Keep it up. Three more . . . two . . . one. All right, you're done."

I collapsed in a heap. I would have groaned if I'd had any air to send through my windpipe.

Joe and Jan packed up their computer and other equipment. Joe would be back in three days, and before leaving, he gave me an assignment: "Write down everything you eat, every day. Don't try to diet, just eat normal foods, but spread it out into six meals throughout the day, and write down the number of calories, protein, and carbs you have in each of the six meals."

"Don't diet?"

He shook his head. "Don't diet. Just eat what you think is healthy, whatever you would normally eat to maintain your weight, not overeating but not necessarily trying to diet either."

"That's it? Just write stuff down? You mean you're not going to put me on some complicated diet and workout scheme that will feel overwhelming and undoable and make me want to give up within forty-eight hours?"

Joe laughed. "Baby steps, Karen, baby steps. Just write down what you eat, and I'll take it from there."

As I closed the front door, I surveyed my surroundings. Everything was back to normal. My living room was just a living room again. My body even felt normal (although I suspected I'd be moaning a different tune the following morning). It was like Rod Serling had returned my life to its regular programming.

Or maybe not.

Something was different, and the difference was in me. The trickle of hope I'd felt on the phone had grown wider and deeper. Now it was more like a pool of hope, maybe even a small lake. It had substance. It was tangible. It was calm and dynamic at the same time.

Something was going to be different this time. I just knew it.

GET A NEW BODITUDE

Questions for Personal Reflection or Group Discussion

• Recall the diets, food plans, exercise routines, and other weight-loss programs you have attempted in the past. Did any of them succeed in changing your body — or the way you feel about your body? Are you still making use of a fitness plan? If so, is it working for you?

• Do you ever feel like you're in a rut?

• Are there any new approaches — counseling, fitness coaching, lifestyle changes, healthier food choices — you keep putting off? What emotions do you feel when you think about embracing new strategies to bring about a lifestyle change?

- Have you reached your turning point? If so, what is different about *this* turning point, in contrast to others in the past?

- Read the following five statements aloud:
  1. I deserve to be healthy and feel beautiful.
  2. There is absolutely no reason why I can't change my body and the way I feel about my body.
  3. I love and accept myself regardless of how much I weigh.
  4. I get to choose what goes into my mouth and onto my hips.
  5. My health and my shape will no longer be controlled by my circumstances, my past, my cravings, or my fears.

They all sound like great statements, don't they? As you were reciting them, did you feel any resistance inside toward any of the statements? Which ones? Did you feel any other unexpected emotions? If so, why do you think that is?

3

Money May Not Grow on Trees, but Change Can Spread Like Wildflowers

MAKING PEACE WITH SMALL CHANGES

Change is organic, like a seedling. It's contagious like laughter. And it's dynamic, not static.

Change is energy. It moves. It impacts everything around it. If you can successfully change one small thing in your life, it will produce ripples and even waves that, before long, jostle other parts of your life into changing. Don't ever underestimate the power of small changes.

I used to despise small changes. I used to think that — in order to lose twenty pounds or stop a bad habit or get control of my finances — I needed to create huge long lists of things I was going to do differently. One January I made a list of resolutions and put it on the refrigerator. It was so long I had to lift the list just to get *into* my refrigerator. I should have realized I was in danger of becoming discouraged by my list rather than motivated.

Sure enough, in the coming weeks, my overzealous list wasn't just an obstacle when it came to getting into the ice cream; it felt like a huge obstacle standing between me and success as well. It represented an overwhelming amount of work. It also delivered a hard blow to my confidence. After all, if my life needed *that* much tweaking, I had to be some kind of loser, right? And if I was *that* big of a mess, why bother even trying to pull my life together?

I'm all for creating and pursuing grand visions for our lives. But sometimes focusing too much on the big picture can feel overwhelming. Sometimes, we're better served by starting small and letting each small success give us the confidence to go a little further, then further still. Imagine each small puff of success as a single burst of steam. Get enough puffs of energy, and before you know it, you've got the momentum of a 150-ton locomotive propelling you down the track.

Whether you need to change your body or just change your opinion of your body, let's look at small changes that will get you moving more and eating healthier. When it comes to loving the skin you're in, you can never go wrong with changes like these.

How Far Can You Possibly Travel on a Treadmill?

I confessed in chapter 1 that I looked in the mirror last year and realized I was fat. This was definitely a case of déjà moo because the same thing happened to me about ten years ago. (Why does weight always sneak up on me like this? Maybe it's because calories are pretty quiet, unless of course you're eating chips.)

Anyway, as soon as this dawned on me, I set a goal to lose fifty pounds in three days. I drove to the gym and launched a mega-mongo workout campaign. Three days later I was not only too sore to move, I was still fat! (I know, it surprised me too. I was so depressed that it took an entire tub of Ben & Jerry's New York Super Fudge Chunk just to lift my spirits enough so I could reach for the Twinkies.)

A week later, admitting that my previous attempt had been too ambitious, I set a kinder, gentler course for myself. I committed to, five days a week, getting dressed in my sweat pants, driving to the gym, and standing on the treadmill.

That was it. Just stand. After that, if I wanted to go home, I could.

Granted, my strategy did not contain any of your normal weight-loss concepts like workouts, food logs, celery sticks, or sweating. Wait, I take that back. Sometimes it involved watching other people sweat, say, for example, if there happened to be someone jogging on the treadmill next to mine. But my own personal sweat was not required.

This was a small change, to be sure. Some people might even argue that it was *too* small. And yet it was a place to start.

What my small change did was eliminate all my excuses. For instance, on days I didn't think I had time to work out, I reminded myself, *But you don't have to work out. All you have to do is drive to the gym and stand on the treadmill. Certainly you can find fifteen minutes for that! And then you can congratulate yourself and enjoy that invigorating feeling of meeting your goal!* And off I'd go to the gym.

On the days when I felt too tired to work out, I pointed out to myself, *But you don't have to work out. All you have to do is drive to the gym and stand on the treadmill. You can't possibly be too tired to just stand there, can you? And then you can give yourself a high five and know that you did it! You met your goal!* And then I would go to the gym.

A lot of days I'd be standing on the treadmill and think, *Well heck, as long as you're here, you might as well turn the thing on.* So I would walk for ten, fifteen, even twenty minutes. Once I got really crazy and broke a sweat. But there were plenty of days when I did nothing but stand on the treadmill and then go home.

What could my exercise in not exercising possibly accomplish? What in the world could it change? Not my body — at least not by much, anyway. Not with the few calories I was burning. But I soon realized that something was being trained and changed, even if it didn't happen to be my body. The first thing getting trained and changed was my mind-set. I stopped asking myself if I was too tired or busy to go to the gym. I didn't even ask myself *if* I would go, but *when.* Within a short time, going to the gym became a nonnegotiable part of my day.

The second thing that was being trained and changed was my schedule. As my trip to the gym became a cornerstone of my day, other tasks and appointments began to fall into place around it. Suddenly finding the time for my daily trek to the treadmill wasn't such a challenge.

My small change had transformed my mind and my habits. With these changes underway, training and changing my body seemed like the natural next step. Over the following ten months, I lost sixty pounds and became as strong, shapely, and toned as I'd ever been. And it began with a very, very, *very* small change.

"EVEN *I* CAN DO THAT!"

I wrote about my "Stand on the Treadmill" strategy in a previous book.[1] Before that book was even released, I got a call from a friend who worked at my publishing company. She'd read my manuscript when it crossed her desk.

She told me, "I've known for years I needed to do something about my health, but the changes I needed to make seemed so overwhelming! Then, four months ago when your manuscript came through the office, I read what you'd done and thought, *That seems simple enough. Even I can do that!* So I started standing on the treadmill. Then I started walking. Then I hired a personal trainer. Now I'm working out five days a week. I've lost thirty-seven pounds, and I haven't felt this good in years!"

To be sure, little changes grow into big changes. But there's something else magical about change, and that is that changes of all sizes love company. They are social creatures, and whenever there's a party (and anytime you're celebrating the success of even a small change, it can feel like a party!), your change is going to want some company.

This is why losing ten pounds suddenly makes you feel like taking up inline skating, or cleaning out your closets, or seducing your husband. Start getting your body whipped into shape, and suddenly getting your kitchen cupboards, checkbook, and even your kids under control won't be far behind.

Whenever I experience success at making a change, I turn into Tony the Tiger. I feel grrrreeeaaat! Suddenly I've got teeth and claws to sink into the next change I've been wanting to tackle. And the change after that. And the one after that.

The best part of this is that we don't have to tackle everything today. We don't have to feel overwhelmed. We don't need to bite off more than we can chew (which, since most of us wouldn't mind losing a few pounds anyway, is probably a good thing).

So if small changes grow into bigger changes, and changes of all sizes travel in herds, what are we waiting for?

To gain the greatest benefit from the social nature of change, I set out to do exactly what Joe had suggested. Or commanded, actually, because you have to ask yourself if it's really a suggestion when someone built like Arnold Schwarzenegger tells you to do something.

On my first day of keeping a food journal, I remembered to write down most of what I ate. The second day I slacked off, skeptical of how helpful my scribbles were going to be. Then Joe e-mailed me a couple of articles about the benefits of keeping a food diary, and suddenly this small change didn't seem like such a trivial exercise any longer. (You can download a sample food journal page from Joe's Web site or from mine, at www.joesbootcamp.com or www.karenlinamen.com.)

Turns out that, according to a six-month study of seventeen hundred overweight men and women, participants who were diligent about keeping a daily food journal lost twice as much weight as participants who kept no records. In fact, according to Jack Hollis of the Kaiser Permanente Center for Health Research and lead author of the study, "Keeping a food diary is one of the most powerful weight-management tools we have."[2]

Twice the weight? Just by writing every day in my food journal? How does that work? I mean, I'm a writer. I write all day. If writing burned that many calories I'd be a size 4 by now.

So apparently, other factors must be at work. And they are.

The first thing I noticed as I began keeping a food diary was that my portions began to shrink. Maybe it's because there's something unsettling about having to make incriminating journal entries such as "Cap'n Crunch cereal, four bowls. Mixing bowls, that is."

The second thing I noticed was that my denial noshing slowed down. Several times a day, as I reached for something I was in the habit of presuming innocent — the abandoned half of a kid's grilled-cheese sandwich, a handful of pretzels, or a chunk of cheddar from the block of cheese I was grating for dinner — it would dawn on me that I'd have to write it down. This, of course, forced me to admit that an abandoned or stolen remnant of food *did* count and *did* contain calories. Admitting this stopped me in my tracks.

Finally, writing everything down gave me

a marker that helped me know when it was time to stop eating for the day. There were times when I'd look at what I'd eaten so far that day and conclude, "That's it. I've eaten my entire day's calories, and now I have to stop for the night." When I first started keeping my journal, there were days I hit this marker by noon. Boy, was that depressing. But soon, I found that by writing everything down, it was easier to pace myself. My food diary helped me remember not to eat my entire day's calories by 10 a.m. It also helped me remember not to swing to the other extreme, going the first half of the day without eating and finding myself transformed by midafternoon into a vacuum cleaner with teeth.

PICK A CHANGE, ANY CHANGE

Going to the gym, even if all we do is stand on a treadmill, is a small but potentially powerful change. So is committing to keep a food diary. There are other small, healthy changes we can make. Is a glass of water small enough?

Everyone's always harping on us to drink eight glasses of water every day, and for good reason. Staying hydrated speeds up your metabolism, flushes impurities out of your body, helps muscles contract more easily (which makes workouts more effective), allows you to feel less hungry, and makes your body less likely to retain water.

Even something as small as going to bed an hour earlier can create a domino effect of healthy benefits. You know how when you're really tired, you sometimes can't stop eating no matter how hard you try? This is because, when you're sleepy, the hormones that are supposed to shut down your appetite aren't doing their job. Apparently sleep is nature's little appetite suppressant, and when we skimp on sleep, we compromise our ability to feel full or know when to say when.

When you sleep less than six hours a night, your body produces less leptin, the blood protein that makes you feel full. And to assist in making sure you weigh more than a refrigerator, your sleep-starved body produces extra grehlin, which makes you want to eat even more. And not more veggies, but more sugar and starches.

If you're still not convinced that skipping sleep can rob you of the hard body you long for, here are some hard numbers: if you average six hours of sleep per night or less, you are 23 percent more likely to be obese than your neighbor who sleeps seven or more hours each night.[3]

NAME YOUR SMALL CHANGE

There's no doubt about it: small changes really can reap big rewards. So what small change are you ready to embrace?

Are you willing to keep a food journal? Go stand on a treadmill? Get to bed one hour earlier? Drink more water? Take the stairs to your office every morning instead of the elevator? Ban mindless snacking at your computer or in front of the television?

We're not talking extreme makeover here. We're talking about a single change. And a small one at that.

Pick one change. Any change. Then watch the momentum roll.

GET A NEW BODITUDE

Questions for Personal Reflection or Group Discussion
- Have you ever made a small change in any area of your life — your health, redecorating a room, making a new friend, starting a business or hobby — that morphed into bigger changes?

- What is one small, healthy change you can decide, today, to incorporate into your life? Write it down.

- What has prevented you in the past from making this change? What will be different this time?

- Have you ever kept a daily food journal? How did that work for you? Why do you think it worked — or didn't work?

- Are you comfortable with making small changes, or do you have an all-or-nothing way of looking at things? If you lean toward all-or-nothing thinking, how do you feel about the idea that, sometimes, one small change may be enough? Does all-or-nothing thinking make the idea of small changes easier or more challenging to embrace?

4
Ever Feel Like Raggedy Ann in a Barbie-Doll World?

MAKING PEACE WITH YOUR OPINION OF YOURSELF

I think women are amazing, I really do. We know how to give birth, change flat tires, run major corporations and small kitchen appliances, raise children, mend broken hearts with chocolate, psychoanalyze our friends' marriages and even our own, cook a holiday turkey, and redecorate an entire house using a single charge card.

So why can't we figure out how to make peace with all the stuff that makes us feel bad about our own bodies? I'm thinking about this as I gather sunscreen, towels, and snacks. I'm getting ready to take my kids to the pool, and I'm feeling . . . well . . . fat.

What does that even mean, "feeling fat"? Fat's not an emotion, it's a condition . . . maybe. Actually, fat is the bodily compound made up of glycerol and fatty acids that stores energy for my muscles, kind of like a battery cell except a lot softer.

But when I say I feel fat, I'm not really feeling like a glycerol-and-fatty-acid battery. What I'm feeling is dissatisfied and disappointed in myself and my shape. I'm probably even feeling disconnected, like there's something preventing me from fully enjoying whatever it is I'm about to do. I'm guessing you've had similar feelings, perhaps while getting ready to go to the pool with your kids, getting dressed up for a night on the town, attending a high-school reunion, or even making love to your husband.

This morning I'm feeling all those things — dissatisfied, disappointed, and disconnected — as I pull open the drawer that holds last year's swimsuits. As I reach for the first candidate, I'm not expecting a happy reunion.

Sometimes I wonder if swimsuits shrink on purpose, if they can be passive aggressive by nature. I'm not a trained swimsuit therapist, but as I pull mine out of the drawer, I can see it has developed a hostile attitude. I would suspect my swimsuit is capable of almost anything — including shrinking two sizes — to get back at me.

Nevertheless, I put it on and look at myself in the mirror. The suit fits, but I'm still not happy. This morning I'm feeling bad about my body, and it's not for any of the reasons I felt bad about my body three weeks ago. Three weeks ago I was in denial, out of shape, and confused about food. These days I'm being proactive. I'm working out with Joe, our muscular personal trainer from chapter 2, and I'm keeping a food diary. I'm feeling stronger. Healthier. I'm even losing weight.

But none of that feels like a victory as I glare at my reflection with a critical eye. This morning, my nemesis isn't food or lethargy or even my scale. This morning, my worst enemy is my opinion of my body.

"I'VE NEVER BEEN HAPPY WITH MY BODY"

The truth is, most of us are unhappy with some aspect of our bodies, and it doesn't matter if we're fat or thin.

Jeacline wrote to me: "I've been on diets since I was seven. I'm not sure how it started, but I always saw myself as fat! Now, it seems ridiculous to me. Seriously! How can 135 pounds be fat? I think back a few years ago and how critical I was of myself. Every inch, every freckle, every little cushion and skin spot was irritating to me. I wanted perfection and didn't even know that I had it already! I had a perfect little body, healthy and strong and completely intact. And I was ungrateful still."

Another woman posted these thoughts on www.experienceproject.com on February 6, 2008: "If I could look in the mirror and like what I see, it would be the best day of my life. I honestly hate myself sometimes. When I walk past a mirror I look away because if I look I'll feel horrible about myself."

Another woman posted resignedly to the same Web site on the same date (though the post has since been removed): "I didn't like [my body] as a teenager; I like it less as a 42 year old woman. Being 5'10" 230 lbs I have never been comfortable with my largeness. Age is hitting now and it's worse, then again no one ever sees it but me so what's the big deal?"

Is there a big deal? How important are our opinions of our own bodies?

Jenny Craig is a body-image consultant. (She does not sell frozen meals; that's a different Jenny altogether.) Jenny is an executive coach and psychotherapist. After years of helping people who had been diagnosed with eating disorders, she has learned a few things about helping people think differently about their bodies.

Jenny tells the story of, early one summer, going swimsuit shopping with a girlfriend. While her friend wriggled in and out of spandex, Jenny watched a group of moms, also shopping for summer apparel, converge on the dressing rooms with several school-aged daughters in tow. As the moms tried on swimsuits, they complained loudly about their hips, their thighs, their butts, their arms, all within earshot of their daughters. Pretty soon Jenny overheard the girls, who were also trying on swimsuits, making similar comments about their own bodies.

Grabbing a bikini off the rack, Jenny threw it on, stepped boldly out of a dressing room, and announced loudly, "Wow! I look fabulous!" She says several of the moms cracked dressing-room doors to see who was making all the commotion and sending a not-so-subtle message.

"Too often women don't think about the true impact of their words," Jenny explains. "They're not thinking about how their words influence their daughters, and they're not aware of how their words are sabotaging their own bodies."

According to Jenny, negative self-talk is one of the reasons people have trouble losing weight. "Negative self-talk increases stress, triggering the body to hold on to stored energy, better known as fat. When we're stressed, our bodies try to use that energy — again, fat — as conservatively as possible, to make it last longer. This is really helpful if you're being chased by a bear, but not particularly helpful when the only thing you need to survive is a trip to the pool."[1] In other words, every time we look at our bodies and stress out, our bodies go into grizzly-bear-survival mode and hang on to our fat even tighter than before. I'm paraphrasing Jenny, but you get the idea.

And not only do our bodies respond to any stress generated by our thoughts or words, our bodies also cooperate with our beliefs. If we tell ourselves we can't lose weight, or that we are destined to wear a size 20 the rest of our lives, our bodies respond as if that spoken belief is set in stone. "The body responds to mental input as if it were physically real," explains Larry Dossey, a physician and advocate for mind-body study. "Images create bodily changes — just as if the experience were really happening. For example, if you imagine yourself lying on a beach in the sun, you become relaxed, your peripheral blood vessels dilate, and your hands become warm, as in the real thing."[2]

According to Jenny Craig, there is a third reason that our beliefs about ourselves matter. Neurological and psychological studies have shown that the brain will take whatever we believe — whether that belief is positive or negative, wrong or right — and search for (and even subconsciously try to create!) evidence that it is true.

Maxwell Maltz, author of the ground-breaking book *Psycho-Cybernetics,* explained why this happens: "Whether we realize it or not, each of us carries about with us a mental blueprint or picture of ourselves. . . . Once an idea or a belief about ourselves goes into this picture it becomes 'true,' as far as we personally are concerned. We do not question its validity, but proceed to act upon it *just as if it were true.*"[3]

In other words, as we degrade our bodies with our words and thoughts, the stress we feel not only triggers our bodies to hang on to fat, but our negative beliefs may actually be telling our bodies how to act. *Plus* our beliefs train our brains to sift through everything we experience, observe, or learn looking for "proof" that we are, indeed, as pathetic as we think we are.

Bottom line: the more we think and speak negatively about ourselves, the more our bodies and brains work to make our false beliefs come true. It's clear that we need to change the things we tell ourselves.

BODY DISSATISFACTION:
NOT JUST SKIN DEEP

Is our opinion of our bodies the real problem? Or does the root of the problem run much deeper, to the core of our opinion of ourselves as *people?* Several nights ago I was pondering this question while driving home after meeting several girlfriends for dinner. We'd just spent a couple of hours talking about events in our lives that had impacted the way we view ourselves. Thinking back on our conversation, I thought, *So what* is *my opinion of me? Not my body, but* me?

Immediately two things came to mind.

I remembered the first Christmas after my husband and I separated. My daughters and I had just decorated our tree — the first live tree I'd purchased in years — and I was sitting on the couch admiring it with my sister, who had dropped over for coffee. About that time my Boston terrier walked over to the tree, lifted his leg, and peed.

Ten minutes later, on my knees with a rag in hand, scrubbing dog urine off the carpet, I confessed, "See? This is the kind of stuff that makes me feel like I'm a failure as a human being."

My sister blinked. "As an *entire* human being?"

I sat on my heels. "Don't you ever feel that way? Like if you were a better person, this kind of stuff wouldn't happen? That you should be able to keep it from happening?"

Michelle stared off for a moment, thinking. Then she said, "No."

I winced. "Really?"

"Dogs pee on trees. There's a tree in your living room. Your dog peed on it. It's nature. Feel bad about the carpet, sure. Get mad at the dog, fine. But it's not you. You didn't do anything wrong. And you know that voice you're hearing, the voice blaming you for not keeping your dog from acting like a dog? We both know whose voice that is." Then she named a certain critical someone who had been a source of disapproval in my life for many years.

The second memory that came to mind was of a conversation that took place one spring when I was living in Texas. Wildflowers were blooming everywhere, and the air felt fertile and alive. Excited, I announced, "I'm going to plant a garden!" The same certain critical someone said, "You can't plant a garden. Everything you plant dies. If you plant a garden, I'm going to rip it out."

I hadn't thought of those two memories for a long time, but they came flooding back on a Colorado summer evening years after the events that spawned them. Similar memories lurked in the shadows. I shook my head to clear them out. I'd remembered enough.

Most of the time, when I ask myself what I think about myself, I give myself rave reviews. After all, I'm compassionate and outgoing and smart and funny. I burn anything I put on a grill, but I make a great banana pudding. I throw a really fun pirate costume party once a year. I'm a great listener and a good friend, even if I do usually show up fifteen minutes late. I'm a pretty savvy entrepreneur and business-woman. I also have this knack for taking seemingly unrelated thoughts and experiences and meshing them into interesting insights about life. I'm a little disorganized, but I'm a lot of fun, and I invest a lot into my relationships. I love, really love, the people in my life. I'm eclectic and interesting. Oh, and did I mention that I'm cute?

I believe all that, I really do. And if you will take an honest inventory of yourself, you will quickly see abilities and strengths and character traits and talent and intelligence and more, all of which set you apart and make you who *you* are. In fact, if you haven't done this recently, take time to look *closely* at yourself before the day is over. Write down what you discover. Make a list of all your strong points. I have no doubt that, just like me, you'll compile a nice little list of what you bring to relationships, family, community, and more.

But — also like me — you may find that along with the good things you believe about yourself, there are darker thoughts, and they have their own power. In my life, I've found that while these darker thoughts may not surface every day, they are always there, swimming just beneath the surface of the sea of me. These are the thoughts that whisper that I'm not good enough or beautiful enough. I'm not desirable. I can't pull my life together and keep it together, whether that means planting a garden or keeping dog urine off the Christmas tree. They're slippery thoughts, showing up at unexpected times, swimming into recesses and places they don't belong.

Sometimes I wonder how these contradictory thoughts can survive together. I wonder why they don't cancel each other out, or why one group doesn't simply swallow up the other. Perhaps you've wondered the same thing about the conflicting thoughts that coexist in your own body of beliefs.

The image that comes to my mind is this:

Imagine you are sitting in a rowboat on a lake, enjoying a glorious summer afternoon. You look out across the water and spot something thick and ominous swimming just below the surface. You see ripples, and sometimes you catch a glimpse of slimy, slithery flesh. You strain your eyes. Eel? Snake? Something even scarier?

You shudder and turn your attention back to your breathtaking surroundings: the expansive sky, the sun's warmth on your skin, reflections on the water, the picnic basket at your feet, and the friend sitting across from you in the gently rocking boat. You focus on these things, but the fact that it's a beautiful day doesn't make the dark shapes go away. The beautiful and the ominous coexist. And you think the ominous shape, living beneath the surface as it does, won't ruin your day. And it doesn't, but you still row a little faster toward shore, and when your friend suggests a swim you recommend a walk instead.

Now I'm going to ask you the same question I asked myself: "Right now, whatever your life is like, what is your opinion of you? Not just your body, but *you?*"

Go ahead. Talk about the gorgeous blue sky and warmth of the sun. Describe the light shimmering on the water and the picnic basket full of good things. Go into detail about all the beautiful things you see when you think about you.

Then take notice of what's under the surface, about the sinister shapes that swim and dart and slither. For just a moment, allow these things to break the surface of the sea that is you, and be honest with yourself about what you see.

WHAT COMES FIRST, THE OPINION OR THE BODY SHAPE?

Why does your opinion of yourself matter — all of it, the beautiful and the sinister? What do your thoughts about your significance and abilities as a woman and human being have to do with the shape of your body?

What comes first? Does your opinion of yourself determine how you treat your body? Or does the shape of your body determine your opinion of yourself?

If you're like me, your body is both source and symptom, cause and effect. Your opinion of yourself influences the shape and health of your body. This is because, when we feel bad about ourselves, eventually our despair or disrespect or even disgust shows up in our bodies. It might look like added weight, or anorexia, or disease. But it shows up.

And as our bodies gain weight or develop eating disorders or disease, it's easy to let our disappointment with our bodies create a deeper dissatisfaction with ourselves as *persons.* By the time we're aware enough of the problem to ask the "cause or effect" question, our opinions have already altered our bodies, which have confirmed our opinions, which have changed our bodies, which have further reinforced our opinions about ourselves.

It's a vicious cycle. But there's good news about vicious cycles. They're not linear, like a river, with a single source you have to dam up if you're going to stop the flow. Cycles are like circles. Interrupt the flow at any point and the whole thing drips to a halt. Which means we have options, lots of options. If you want to stop the circle, start making changes anywhere you want.

Begin by working on your body. Or by working on the way you speak and think about your body. Or begin by working on your opinion of yourself as a human being. Eventually you'll probably need to work on all of the above, but to begin making changes, you can start anywhere you want. The choice is yours.

As I stand in front of my mirror wearing last year's swimsuit and frowning at my body, I think I know what I need to do next. I've already begun to interrupt the cycle by working on my body — my workouts with Joe and my food journal testify to that. And if you've been coming along with me on this journey, you've probably been working on your body too. So maybe now is a good time to tackle the vicious circle from a different direction. Maybe now is a good time to take a look at some of our beliefs about *us.*

Where exactly are we getting the belief that we're not good enough, pretty enough, or smart enough, or that we're subhuman if we can't keep dog pee off a Christmas tree or plants alive in a garden? And more important, what can we do about it?

Let's figure it out together in chapter 5.

GET A NEW BODITUDE

Questions for Personal Reflection or Group Discussion
- Deep down, how do you feel about your body? What is your opinion of yourself as a woman and a human being? Can

---

you identify any connections between the two?

- Think of recent comments you have made about your body. Were they mostly positive or mostly negative?

- Do you feel you have developed your view of yourself on your own? Or are your opinions being influenced by painful experiences from your past or negative opinions and comments of others?

- What do you think about Jenny Craig's comments in this chapter that negative self-talk raises our stress levels and can also prompt our brains to find ways to support negative opinions of ourselves?

5

Tony Danza's Not the Boss of You

MAKING PEACE WITH TAKING CHARGE

Let's face it. You and I are bombarded with negative messages from society, from the media, from advertising, sometimes from religion, and even from loved ones and friends. Oddly, we accept and trust these negative messages, perhaps because we think outsiders know us better than we know ourselves.

But do they *really?*

Granted, no one is completely objective about her own life. We're too hard on ourselves in some areas, while we too easily let ourselves off the hook in other areas. But we're not *entirely* in la-la land when it comes to assessing our strengths and weaknesses. I mean, who else has lived in your skin every second of every day of every year of your life? Only one person, *you!* So give yourself some credit for being a good judge of character when you're taking a personal inventory.

There is a second reason we get down on ourselves: entire industries have grown up around keeping us dissatisfied. The most blatant — and pervasive — of these is the advertising industry. Running a close second is the fashion industry.

When these groups and others succeed in making us feel like we don't measure up — bingo! — they profit. So the next time you're watching television or reading a magazine article and get that empty feeling about yourself, remember that the input you are receiving was not created for your personal benefit. People came up with that stuff to advance their cause or make money at your expense. Advertisers are successful *only* when they convince you that you are less than good enough *unless* you buy the product or service they are selling. You need their cosmetics, jewelry, hair gel, sexy jeans, luxury ride . . . and then, just maybe, you will measure up. But measure up to what?

Think about the insanity of women's fashion and the annual introductions of the new spring and fall lines. Just watch one of those shows on television, in which eerily tall and frighteningly thin supermodels strut, loose-jointedly, down a runway wearing garments that no woman in her right mind would be seen in. Have you ever, even once, known a woman older than twenty whose dimensions match a runway model's, or who has ever, even in a fit of temporary madness, worn clothing that resembles what you see modeled in a fashion show?

The fashion industry is not normal. Yet as unreliable and bizarre as the industry is, it still makes us believe lies about ourselves.

Need another example? How about the nation's leading sports magazine? Every winter, *Sports Illustrated* releases its swimsuit issue, completely ignoring the fact that "swimsuit" is not a recognized sport in any nation on earth. It's impossible to win an Olympic medal in "swimsuit." But that doesn't stop this magazine from subjecting us to their January swimsuit edition, an annual tradition that is the inspiration for pity-party binges and resulting weight gain for nonsupermodel women everywhere.

WHY WE BUY THE LIES

I get why we're unhappy with our bodies and, by extension, with who we are. I really do. And while I agree these are factors that we, as a society, need to address, I think there's more to the story. I believe the number one reason you and I end up with tarnished beliefs about ourselves and our bodies is that we're not *intentional* about creating opinions of ourselves that are worth having. We're intentional about so many other things, so why can't we invest in ourselves with the same level of attention?

I used to be intentional about garage sales. Every Friday I grabbed the paper, hit the classifieds, and made a map showing the locations of all the garage sales I wanted to shop at the next morning.

I know a woman who is intentional about department-store sales the day after Thanksgiving. She gets ready the night before, setting out comfortable clothes and shoes, a big shopping bag, and an arsenal of credit cards. She gathers all the ads detailing all the sales at all the stores she wants to visit. She knows where she's going to park, which door she'll be stalking at 7 a.m., and which registers tend to have the shortest lines.

I know a woman who is intentional about her body. She works out every day, shuns carbs, nixes artificial sweeteners, and stocks her fridge with veggies. She even creates a kinder, gentler environment for her body by avoiding toxic household cleaners, cleaning her windows with vinegar and washing her clothing with biodegradable detergent. And heaven help the unsuspecting person who lights up a cigarette in her presence!

My sister Michelle is intentional about the

way she parents her daughter and step-daughters. Her intention is to give Gabriella, Abby, and Molly important life skills in every category, and she exposes these lucky girls to a carefully thought out array of books, classes, experiences, and even reward systems. From sports and social graces, to values and spirituality, Michelle really thinks about the things she wants to teach her daughters. She creates strategies and makes them happen.

My friend Ilene is intentional about the way she spends her money. After twenty-five years of frugal living, she and her husband, Tom, live on a paid-off ranch and drive paid-off cars. They garden. They raise chickens. They live in an energy-efficient, earth-bermed ranch house that Tom built from scratch. And they've done it all while bringing in a combined income of roughly twenty-five thousand dollars a year for much of their married life. This kind of financial stability doesn't happen by accident; it happens on purpose.

I don't know what you're intentional about. Perhaps it's the way you decorate your house, or run a business, or relate to your husband or your kids. When it comes to certain things, you and I seem to understand that the results we crave will not evolve by chance. We understand that we can't just "go with the flow" and expect to reach the destination of our dreams. Instead, we embrace a vision, create a plan, prepare to follow that plan, and then judge everything that comes into our lives accordingly, making decisions to pass or pursue opportunities depending on whether they'll move us closer to our vision.

And yet when it comes to the way we think about our bodies or even the way we think about ourselves, we can be pretty aimless, simply drifting with whatever tides and currents come our way.

What does aimless look like? *Aimless* is wallowing in self-pity. Reliving old hurts. Rehearsing that feeling of "not good enough," playing with it like the sore in your mouth that you caress with your tongue over and over again. And when the currents created by society, past rejection, hurtful comments, or unhealthy relationships send you drifting downstream, *aimless* is allowing yourself to be swept over the waterfall to crash on the rocks below. In contrast, being *intentional* means locking your gaze on the horizon you have chosen, setting your jaw, and rowing as hard and steady as you can to reach a safe shore.

WHAT DOES INTENTIONAL LOOK LIKE?

What does it mean to be intentional about forming an accurate understanding of our bodies and ourselves? It starts with taking charge and realizing that we, alone, are the gatekeepers of our beliefs. It demands that we consciously choose what messages to accept — and what messages to reject — and it doesn't matter if those messages come from billboards, *Sports Illustrated,* childhood experiences, ex-boyfriends or husbands, moms in dressing rooms whining about their flabby arms, or even ourselves.

Several years ago a young woman told me an amazing story. Here's what she related: "When I was fifteen, maybe sixteen, I used to feel bad about my body. I hated wearing bathing suits and I hated wearing shorts. Seriously, I thought I was the ugliest person ever born. As I became more conscious of the thoughts I was having about myself, one day I realized there wasn't a woman I knew who deserved to think about herself like that."

Then her mom gave her some great advice, suggesting that the young woman take an objective look at herself, literally. Acting on the advice, every time she got out of the shower, this young woman would stand naked in front of a mirror and look at her body — really look at it — and begin to speak truth about her body. Speaking the truth gradually counteracted the lies she'd been telling herself. She explained it to me like this:

Every time I got out of the shower, I stood in front of a mirror and told myself how beautiful I was while looking at my naked body, so I would begin to associate the words with what I was seeing. I'd start at my feet and say, "Oh! You have the most beautiful feet!" Then my legs, my hips — all the parts I was particularly self-conscious about — all the way up to my head.

I didn't just try to say the words, I also made a decision to interact with that truth in as many ways as I could. I spoke the truth aloud with my mouth. I looked in the mirror and watched my lips forming the words. I listened to the words with my ears. Sometimes I would even write the words down on paper. I purposely tried to involve as many of my senses as I could.

It changed the way I view myself and my ability to love myself and accept myself. And you know what? I'm the exact same weight that I was back when I wouldn't wear a bathing suit. Now I'm confident, and I love my body and wouldn't trade it, even though it's the exact same body I had when I hated myself.

NOW THAT'S INTENTIONAL

Isn't that a wise woman? And what a wise mom she has. Why can't I be more like this young woman or her mom?

Oh, wait. That young woman is my daughter, Kaitlyn. Which would make her mom . . . me. Which makes my own insecurities about my body and myself rather ironic, don't you think? I'm thinking maybe it's time I tried following the advice I apparently gave Kaitlyn.

Being intentional about the messages we choose to accept — even from the woman who is staring back at us in the mirror — can make all the difference in the world. And I'm not just talking about messages about our bodies. The messages we choose to accept about our value and significance as women and as human beings are just as important, and maybe even more so.

Because it's been a few years since Kaitlyn told me this story, I called her about twenty minutes ago and asked her to tell me her story again. I wanted to make sure I had the details right. She told me the story, and it was just like I've written it here. Except she left out one part. After she finished retelling the story, I asked, "What about the part where the whole thing was my idea? I mean, I'm not trying to take credit here or anything, but it's a funny twist to my chapter."

"Oh, that," Kaitlyn said nonchalantly. "I made that part up."

I blinked. "What?"

"I said I made it up."

"What? When? And why?"

"When I told you about it a couple of years ago, I made up the part about how it was your idea. It was a time in my life when I was afraid other people would think my ideas were dumb; so even when I had a good idea, I always said it was someone else's. Don't you remember? The first time I told you about my mirror exercise and told you it was your idea, you said, 'No it wasn't.' And I said, 'Yes, it was.' And you said, 'Huh, that's funny, I don't even remember it.'"

I know the conversation she's talking about, and she's right: I didn't remember giving her that advice. Because I didn't give it to her!

I started to laugh. Hard.

Kaitlyn said, "Hey, if you want, for your book you can say it was your idea, especially since I worked so hard to convince you that it was. It doesn't matter to me."

I was still laughing. "Are you kidding? You're brilliant. The affirmations you came up with, and the way you figured out to interact with the truth with all your senses, it's brilliant, baby. You are an incredibly wise young woman. There's no way in a million years I'd take credit for your idea."

Besides, it makes a much better story the way it really happened, don't you agree?

Before Kaitlyn and I got off the phone, I just had to ask. "So why now? Why are you ready now to say that you had a good idea?"

"I'm more confident now."

"Did accepting your body have anything to do with accepting yourself in other ways too? You know, like realizing not only do you have great feet, but you're capable of great ideas too?"

"Yeah, it really did."

I guess it goes back to that vicious cycle. Except maybe it's not so vicious after all. Improve what you think about yourself, and you will be in a great position to improve how you feel about your body. And as you feel better about your body, you may find your confidence growing in other areas as well.

Without a doubt, there is a mystery and beauty about the way our bodies, minds, and spirits are connected. We really are fearfully and wonderfully made.

GET A NEW BODITUDE

Questions for Personal Reflection or Group Discussion

- Could you do what my daughter did? Could you stand naked in front of a mirror and describe your body, part by part, as being special and beautiful? Why or why not? What emotions do you think such an exercise would evoke in you?

- Are there other steps — in addition to positive affirmations — that you can take to change the way you think about your body? Listen to what a woman named Anne decided to do: "I found pictures of plus-size models and looked at them a lot, so I could normalize what I saw in the mirror. Then, whenever I felt insecure about my weight, I would think,

---

I am what a woman looks like. When I did look in the mirror, I made sure to think about how awesome it is that my body could do whatever I wanted it to, that I'm healthy, and how fabulous that was. After about six months, my insecurity just sort of melted away." Could you do what Anne did? Why or why not?

• List your top seven feelings about your body and yourself. Read the list and give it careful thought. Are there any that you would like to change? If so, what is your first step in changing them?

6

If We Are What We Eat, Does That Mean I'm Fast, Cheap, and Easy?

MAKING PEACE WITH FOOD

One week Trainer Joe and I planned something a little different. We decided he'd come over in the morning and put me through my workout paces, then I'd make us some lunch, and we'd spend an hour working on a weight-loss article for the local newspaper.

That morning I scanned my pantry for options. Imagine the pressure! What kind of meal do you serve to a personal trainer? I pulled my hand back from the extra cheesy mac and cheese and the bag of Oreos. Instead, I readied a pot of long grain rice, some steamed yellow squash, and baked chicken.

After a killer workout, Joe began packing away his equipment while I headed to the kitchen. When he walked in a few minutes later, I had our plates filled and waiting at the table.

"Wow! Smells great!" he said, and then he

began to laugh. "Um, remind me, in a future session, to talk about portion sizes."

I blinked. "Why?"

Turns out I'd filled his plate with roughly four times what a healthy portion of chicken, rice, and veggies should look like. Apparently a healthy portion would have been half a cup of cooked rice, one cup of veggies, and a piece of chicken about the size of Joe's palm.

"But you're a big guy," I countered, "shouldn't your portions be bigger?"

"Nope." He told me he tries to stick with healthy-size portions, and that if he's still hungry in half an hour he simply eats an extra small meal. "It takes twenty minutes for our stomachs to tell our brains that we've eaten. So even though I'm a big guy, I give each mini-meal plenty of time to do its job before chasing it with more food."

BETTER LATE THAN NEVER

Until now, my philosophies about food have pretty much toggled back and forth between "eat whenever you're hungry, happy, sad, or bored" and "when you want to lose weight, stop eating." Oh, and then there's "I brake for chocolate." And on the days Joe works me really hard, I could go for a bumper sticker that says "Personal trainer in trunk."

So all this other stuff — like protein servings the size of your hand — are major paradigm shifts for me. And the shifts get even wilder.

After lunch, Joe and I sat down in my office and created an outline for a newspaper article. He had agreed to continue training me in exchange for my writing some articles for him, so I was happy to be working on this story. But I was also happy because, as we talked, I discovered a whole new way to think about food.

We talked about when to eat, what to eat, and even how to eat. From what I gathered, making peace with food boils down to asking ourselves six important questions before we reach for anything to eat.

1. "Am I eating for fuel?"

Consider these restaurant slogans: "Come hungry. Leave happy" (IHOP). "Food is love" (Summer Shack seafood restaurants). "Good food . . . good feelings" (Village Inn).

In these and many other ways, you and I have been conditioned to associate food with emotions and entertainment rather than fuel and nutrition. And yet, as a general rule, the purpose of food is to fuel your body. (I know! It was news to me too!)

Before you or I put anything in our

mouths, we need to know why we're reaching for whatever it is we're reaching for: Is it for fuel? If not — if we're eating to meet a different need — then we need to ask whether food is really the best solution we can come up with, or is there something else we can do to meet that need?

That's not to say there's no place for a little social noshing. From birthday cake and Sunday dinners to backyard potlucks and lingering conversations in romantic restaurants, there's no denying the social benefits of sharing a meal together. The question is, how can we enjoy the benefits without making our bodies pay the price?

Here are some ideas:

- Ask yourself if you're "eating for fuel" and try to stick with healthy portions of healthy food.
- Spend less time eating and more time focusing on mingling and enjoying the people around you.
- Don't show up at a party or social gathering famished. Eat a healthy meal *before* you go to the event. No one will mind that you spend less time at the buffet table and more time visiting with them!

2. "When was the last time I ate?"

While Joe and I were working on the outline, my sister Michelle dropped by. When we told her what we were working on, she got her thoughtful look. You could almost see the wheels turning.

Then she said, "Okay, Joe, maybe you can give me some advice. I work nights as a police dispatcher. I get off work at seven in the morning, drive half an hour home, and am usually heading to bed around eight. But by then, after being up all night, I'm hungry, tired, and sometimes stressed about stuff in my personal life. Sometimes it's almost like I'm in a fog. So I eat. Actually, I go to bed eating. I eat peanuts and junk food in bed and read a book until I fall asleep. And I'm packing on the pounds."

"When you're going to bed at eight in the morning," Joe asked her, "how long has it been since you've eaten?"

"My lunch break is around 4 a.m., so I guess it's been around four hours."

Joe had it figured out. "You're hungry because it's time for your body — which needs fuel every two to three hours — to have another meal. You're experiencing true hunger. Try this: As soon as you're off work — before you leave the building or while driving home — have a protein shake. By the time you get home, your stomach will have had time to let your brain know you've eaten something and you won't be as hungry. True hunger can be a natural lead-in to emotional eating. You start eating for legitimate reasons, then keep eating even when you're full because your brain hasn't gotten the news yet. By the time you feel full, you're actually overstuffed *and* you're on a roll and into the emotional eating segment of the experience!"

Joe also suggested that Michelle — starting immediately — create a habit of *only* eating at the kitchen table, nowhere else in the house. "If you get home and you're still hungry — and it's been half an hour or so since the protein shake — then make yourself a healthy snack and enjoy it at the table. The rules of this new habit are: Set a nice table. Prepare your food. Sit down. Eat slowly and don't just mindlessly shovel it in. Now you're ready for bed."

Michelle and I both benefited from Joe's advice. And perhaps you can too. The next time *you* find yourself reaching for junk food, ask yourself how long it has been since you last ate. If it has been more than two or three hours, it's time to give your body what it really wants, which is a healthy meal. Then stop eating for at least twenty minutes to give your brain time to get the news.

3. "Am I sabotaging myself by using big dishes?"

A big plate or bowl invites a big serving. Think about the size of your dinnerware, then shift to using smaller plates. Buy a dinner set that's a little smaller or use a salad plate. You'll still be eating the food you like, but it'll just naturally be a smaller portion.

I've started eating some of my meals from a mug! Not even a big mug, but just a small coffee-cup-size mug. It seems to be about the right size for a healthy serving of most foods, which more often than not translates into about a half cup of whatever it is I'm eating, such as rice and beans, or yogurt and a little granola. I'm trying to limit my six daily meals to around two hundred fifty calories each, which also helps me figure out how much to eat.

4. "Am I taking enough time to really enjoy my food?"

Since we love food so much, you'd think we'd slow down enough to really savor a good meal. But we live in a fast-paced world, where the temptation is to inhale our food while multitasking or right before we run out the door. The problem is, there is a twenty-minute delay between mealtime and the time our brains know we've eaten — so we won't feel full for about a half hour. If we eat in a hurry or amid too many distractions, it's too easy to shovel in way more food than we need. Then, thirty minutes later, we get that stuffed-to-the-gills, "why in the world did I eat all that?" feeling.

Solution? Leave the television and computer, and eat at the table, where you can stay aware of what and how much you're eating. And s-l-o-w d-o-w-n. Put your fork down between bites. Chew. Savor. Enjoy. Joe says, "If you really want to eat slower, try eating with your left hand if you're right handed, and vice versa. Just don't stab yourself in the cheek."

5. "Am I eating the right kinds of carbs?"

We need carbs. Don't let anyone tell you otherwise. In fact, carbs are our bodies' first preferred source of fuel. But all carbs are not created equal. Good carbs — whole grains and colorful fibrous fruits and veggies such as red and yellow peppers, spinach, and yams — are rich in fiber. These are the good guys.

Then there are carbs that are highly processed, like white bread, rice, bagels, white tortillas. Processed carbs such as these turn to sugar quickly in your bloodstream. These are the bad guys.

How do you know if you're eating the right kind of carbs? Follow these rules:

- Don't eat white or beige. Fiber-rich carbs tend to be darker — like whole wheat or rye breads — or colorful like yams.
- Follow the 10-2 rule. Look at the nutritional information. For every 10 grams of carbs there should be at least 2 grams of fiber.
- Avoid high-fructose corn syrup at all costs because your body has a hard time processing it. Unfortunately, it's a cheap filler found in most processed foods. Even a lot of whole-grain products are made with high-fructose corn syrup. Instead, try breads made from sprouted live grains such as Ezekiel Bread that don't use high-fructose corn syrup for filler or flavor.

6. "What will I be doing in the next three hours?"

Okay, this one was a real eye-opener for me. Joe told me that, since carbs give me fuel for movement, I should eat carbs only when I deserve them, meaning if I'm going to be moving around and will need energy, or if I've just had an intense workout. He said, "Most of us are sedentary, sitting in office chairs, e-mailing instead of walking around talking to people. We either stay at our desks and work through the lunch break to get more stuff done, or we have a huge lunch with co-workers and then go back to sitting at our desks. With all that not-moving, why do we even need carbs? Carbs fuel your body for movement."

Bottom line: If you're not going to be moving in the next three hours, you don't need carbs. Fill up on proteins and non-starchy vegetables like celery instead. To help make this a habit, Joe suggests the "three-hour rule." Before eating anything, ask yourself: "What am I going to be doing in the next three hours?" And fill up accordingly. Eat according to what your body's going to need in the next several hours.

MAKING PEACE WITH MY PANTRY

Changing your approach to food is not easy, but it's simple. Here's what I've learned so far:

- Keep a food diary.
- Eat six small meals per day.
- Limit portion size. A healthy portion

of a complex carb like brown rice or a sweet potato is about half a cup. A healthy portion of vegetables is about a cup. A healthy portion of lean meat is about the size of my palm.

- Check the clock. Wait at least twenty minutes before reaching for a second helping, because it takes that long for your stomach to tell your brain that you're not starving anymore.
- Enjoy your food. Sit down at the table and eat slowly.
- Match food to your activity level. Choose carbs carefully, and save most of your carbs for when you know you'll be active in the next three hours.

All of this sounds simple, but it fails to answer one question: When do I eat the Oreos, or the Doritos, or the pecan-praline ice cream? Or any of the other goodies in my fridge and pantry that don't seem to have a readymade place in the New Food Script that Joe is writing for me? I'm still working on that one. Maybe I'll ask Joe next week. At the moment, all I can tell you for sure is that none of my junk-food favorites seem to have a starring role in the daily food drama, at least not the way Joe's rewriting the script.

Then again, maybe that's okay. These were always troublesome characters anyway. Not to mention drama kings and queens. Maybe now — with my junk-food divas receiving only bit parts and cameos once in a while — we'll all be happier. Maybe my daily food drama won't feel so drama-ridden. Maybe it can turn into something else entirely. Something a little lighter.

A romantic comedy might be nice.

GET A NEW BODITUDE

Questions for Personal Reflection or Group Discussion

• With Joe's recommended portion sizes in mind, do you suspect you've been eating too much? How do you feel about the amount of food you eat — at meal-time, plus snacks?

• When you think of eating smaller portions, what happens? Do you sense panic, resignation, sadness, or hopelessness? Anger? Anxiety? What about either of these: "No way! I'll be too hungry!" or "Nobody's going to tell *me* how much to eat!" What emotions or thoughts are rising to the top?

• How hard would it be for you to go one month without eating any junk food?

7

THE SEVEN HABITS OF WOMEN WHO KNOW HOW TO CHOOSE THEIR HABITS

MAKING PEACE WITH HABITUAL BEHAVIORS

Joe's advice to my sister made perfect sense. Michelle was working the night shift and arriving home at seven in the morning. Joe suggested she drink a protein shake before she left work, so that by the time she arrived home, her brain would register that her hunger had been satisfied. Making this small change helped keep her from snacking at home, eating in bed, and eating too much just before she fell asleep.

Eating is something we do because it's necessary for survival, of course. But it's also something we do out of habit, often without thinking. So whether we work the night shift or day shift, or work at home, or earn our pay doing physical labor or sitting at a computer, we need to form healthy habits that make eating much more intentional.

A habit is usually a very simple thing that produces incredible results, so here is one we all need to adopt: at no time should we eat anywhere but at the kitchen table, or the break-room table if we're at the office. Choosing this habit and practicing it can bring our mindless eating to a screeching halt.

But here's the rub. A habit produces great results only if we stick with it. And really, when it comes down to it, aren't habits at the root of a lot of our issues with the way we feel about our bodies? With the right eating habits, we could have shapelier bodies. With the right exercise habits, we could have stronger bodies. With the right thinking habits, we could have healthier opinions of ourselves.

Sometimes we can identify the habits we need to change. Sometimes we can even change them. Very often, however, our habits get the best of us, sticking around as stubbornly as jokes about Billy Ray's mullet.

I think I'm onto something. I may have figured out a way to live life unhindered by bad habits. I can honestly say that I have great habits, that every single habit is exactly what I want and is empowering me to succeed in achieving my chosen goals . . . if my goals boil down to being overdrawn at the bank, overweight in my swimsuit, and overwhelmed by all the clutter in my house.

Don't laugh. Why can't these be my goals? After all, when it feels as if it's too hard to change our habits to match our goals, why not change our goals to match our habits?

Voilà! Instant success.

So why don't I feel like celebrating?

CREATURES OF HABIT

Habits are the little anchors that tether us to the lifestyles to which we've become accustomed. If we're lucky (or smart), our habits are anchoring us to lifestyles that we love. If we have been careless, our habits may be anchoring us to lifestyles we wish we could trade in for something a little more rewarding and enjoyable.

People talk a lot about how to change habits. In fact, I'm one of those people, having written a book titled *Only Nuns Change Habits Overnight: 52 Amazing Ways to Master the Art of Personal Change.* But right now, the first thing I want to change is the word *change.* Let's change it to *choose.* Obviously this wouldn't have worked at all for my previous book. That's because no one would have bought a book that promised "52 amazing ways to master the art of personal choose."

Be that as it may, in this chapter the new wording will work just fine. In fact, it's going to be great, because I want to talk about the seven habits of women who know how to choose their habits. Choose, not change. The word choice is crucial, because sometimes "change" feels daunting, especially when we're talking about deeply ingrained habits like how we eat, how often we exercise, and the opinions we hold about our bodies and ourselves. When we talk about changing these habits, it can feel like double the work, as if we have to kill the old habit even as we embrace a new one.

But think about the freedom we gain when we can *choose* . . . Ahh, that feels like something altogether different, doesn't it? As if the slate has been wiped clean and all that's left for us to do is point an index finger at the brand-new collection of habits we'd love to own. Choose the best new habits and it's a done deal.

Choosing makes me think of salivating in front of the display counter at the See's Candies in Downey, California, where I grew up. I'd ride my bike there from my house on Samoline Street, past the Sav-On Drugs and the Bob's Big Boy Restaurant, back when checkered-pants Bob — big boy that he was — still waved customers inside for a juicy Big Boy cheeseburger and fries.

But I digress.

(Boy, did I ever! How did I start out talking about choosing healthier habits and end up at See's Candies on my way to enjoy a Big Boy's cheeseburger? Must be getting close to lunchtime.)

Anyway, that's what the word *choose* makes me think of. As if it really is within my power to decide. After all, some things I can change (like my hair color), and some things I can't (like the national debt). But choosing, that's something that feels doable.

THE SEVEN HABITS OF WOMEN WHO KNOW HOW TO CHOOSE THEIR HABITS

So how hard is it to consciously choose the habits that will shape your life? Is there a special set of required skills or traits? Does it involve something that is difficult to acquire, like a leprechaun or a genie?

I've identified seven things common to women who are successful at choosing their habits. Women who choose their habits with intention and success understand the power of each one. And by liberally applying the seven dynamics to whatever new habit you want to embrace, you can reap a new and improved life.

1. Perspective

What do you see when you look at the new habit you're choosing? Do you see it as something to dread? Or do you see this new habit as something that, as soon as you make it part of your daily repertoire, will be an enjoyable part of your day?

If you choose a new habit designed to achieve a goal that you feel you've already failed at, you'll lose steam right from the start. So look at your end goal from a new angle. Instead of tackling the same ten pounds that have defeated you before, choose to do something new and inspiring. (How about this for a new goal: "Forget losing weight — been there done that! My goal is, by the end of the summer, to build up my stamina until I can jog six miles without stopping or needing CPR!")

How you look at choosing a new habit — whether you see it as blessing or bane — will determine whether you embrace it boldly or hold it at arm's length like yesterday's Limburger.

2. Preparation

A new habit needs all the help it can get. It's like a baby who grows sturdy legs quickly, but at the beginning, while it's still crawling and learning how to walk, you've got to do your share to make things as easy for the habit as you can. So protect your toddling habits by habit-proofing your house.

Have you chosen a habit that will help you eat healthier? Help the habit by not keeping dangerous junk food in an accessible place like your pantry or, actually, anywhere in your house. Get rid of it immediately, maybe sooner.

Does your new habit involve getting up at the crack of dawn and hitting the gym? Then protect that little habit by turning off the television or computer at a reasonable hour and getting enough sleep, so when your alarm goes off at 5:45 a.m., you don't fling it violently across the room and kill someone.

Do you want to think uplifting, positive thoughts about yourself and your life? Then put away sharp objects like that framed photo of Mr. Ex who broke your heart and left you feeling about as desirable as the smelly leftover you found in the fridge, hiding in orange Tupperware. And you know that CD the Ex burned for you, with all his favorite sappy songs? Return the favor and BURN IT.

Now that you've made your life a safer habitat for your fledgling habits, continue preparing for success. Be proactive. Fill your fridge with healthy alternatives, or lay out your running shoes and sweat pants the night before, or stock your bedside reading stack with encouraging books, and your iPod with motivating messages and music.

3. Interruption

Yes, I realize this doesn't start with P. But it's important, so work with me here.

Nighttime is hard for me. I often find myself trying to fall asleep while wrestling with worries about life: career issues, kid issues, finances, relationships, health issues, matters of weight and beauty, and even that court date I missed last month related to a speeding ticket. (If this chapter ends abruptly, mid-sentence, you'll know the long arm of the law has caught up with me.) As long as I'm lying awake counting my problems, sometimes I picture them wearing sheepskins, but it hasn't put me to sleep yet. With all these nagging dilemmas running roughshod in my brain, it's easy to feel discouraged about my body, myself, and even my future.

If you see yourself in my description, choose a new habit to embrace hope whenever you can. Sounds great, doesn't it? But what does that look like in real life? When it's late at night and you're kept awake by old, scary worries and consumed by dark anxieties — what can you do?

In those moments when your old habits are fully operational and the new habit you have chosen feels temporarily out of commission, the least you can do is toss a monkey wrench in the gears of the old habit! Do something — anything! — to get yourself out of the well-worn rut of your old habit. Whether you're lying awake counting problems in sheep's clothing, scooping yourself a huge bowl of ice cream, or berating yourself for how you look in a swimsuit, interruption is your friend!

Jump up and take the dog for a walk, turn on some rock and roll, or — here's a fun one! — seduce your husband! Put in a load of laundry or pick up an encouraging book or magazine. Play a game of solitaire. Turn on the Cartoon Network. Drive to the all-night supermarket, and pick up tomorrow's newspaper while the ink's still wet.

You don't have to rev up the engine of your new habit right now. Just slam on the brakes and bring the old one to a screeching halt.

4. Partners

Women who successfully choose (and use!) good habits understand the power of partnership. You can grab a walking partner, get a mentor, register for a weight-loss program, work out with a fitness trainer, hire a life coach, or visit a psychologist. I've done every one of these things. They're good things.

You can also simply hang out with people who are already succeeding at the new habit you've chosen for yourself. I do this and love it. I want to be intentional about choosing habits that will grow my skills as a writer and speaker, so I hang out with other writers and speakers. One group of about thirty writers meets monthly at a café in an eclectic neighborhood on the outskirts of Colorado Springs. If you're in the area on the fourth Thursday evening of any given month, stop in.[1] Guillarmo, the café's owner, makes panini to drool over. And his chocolate-covered coconut Cucuroons are out of this world. (Oops, sorry. Another unfortunate illustration in a book about making peace with our waistlines!)

Another, more intimate group of writers meets at my house every four to six weeks. Mike, Andy, Laura, Beth, Blythe, Steve, Keith, and Gaylyn are priests, role models, and cheerleaders rolled into one — or eight, as the case may be. (You should see Mike, Andy, Keith, and Steve in short skirts and pompoms.) We've been meeting for four years, and no one misses a meeting. It's better than therapy. Best of all, it's inspiring to see what each one has managed to accomplish in that period of time. Goals that felt like pipe dreams forty-eight months ago — for each of us — have come true. And I have no doubt that part of the transformation from dream to reality has come from sharpening our good habits on the whetstone of friendships with like-minded souls.

5. Persistence

Women who successfully choose their habits understand the power of persistence.

I had a good cry last night. There are some areas of my life I just can't seem to get right no matter how fast I peddle. Curled up in bed, I wept and wrote out my frustrations in my journal. Working out with Joe and eating right, I managed to lose sixteen pounds — then had an emotional week and found seven of those lost pounds at the bottom of an ice cream carton. (Several cartons, actually, but who's counting?) I'm late on a writing deadline. I bounced a few more checks. I'm jealous of my sisters because they're skinnier than I am. I just broke up with someone I really liked because . . . Well, perhaps that's a story for another chapter. Old hurts and wounds from when I was married flare up now and then, and last night they were inflamed and throbbing.

Then, earlier that evening, I was standing on a ladder putting something away on a high shelf next to a ceiling fan (and please don't ask why I didn't turn off the fan. I don't *know* why I didn't turn it off), and one of the blades cracked my finger — hard — and for the next hour, holding a bag of frozen peas against my swollen knuckle, I wondered if it might be broken. Worst of all, my roots are showing, and I can't see my hairdresser till next week.

I felt like giving up. Last night I did give up.

Sometimes, in my journal, I write letters to God, and last night was one of those occasions.

Lord, I feel so sad right now . . . like everything is for naught, like I strive and strive and nothing is coming together like I envision. Some days I feel so weary. And I'm stressed and eating! I'm so discouraged about weight and food. Lord, please help me focus and prioritize

103

and get things done. And eat right, too, not taking it out on my body . . . I'm so tired, really tired, of everything feeling like it's uphill. Is this what it all amounts to, really? My heart hurts. It's like there's a huge hurt in there. I work so hard to overcome it in so many ways . . . lately I feel as if it is winning . . . But maybe that's okay. Maybe I don't even care anymore.

This morning I washed the dried tears off my face and put on my running shoes. I hit the dirt roads near my house by 6:30 and got to watch the sun come up. I came home and Bisselled my carpets, changed my sheets, and put on a pot of soup. While I was cleaning my room, I found a picture of my mom and dad. It's on my Web site (www.karenlinamen.com) if you'd like to see it. They're looking at a motorcycle, and they're holding each other like they're love-drenched newlyweds. Married fifty years and counting. I taped it to my mirror as a reminder that, yes, true love exists. Then I sat down and wrote eight pages toward my deadline.

You're trying to reinvent your life. Some days you'll feel like giving up. Some days you will give up.

That's okay. You have my permission. Go ahead. Give up.

But just until morning.

6. Pats on the Back

Women who are successful at choosing their habits know the power of praise. And if no one else is giving it to you, give it to yourself! Sometimes praise is found in glowing words. Tell yourself, "You go, girl!" Say it with a high-five in front of a mirror.

Sometimes we praise ourselves by not poo-pooing praise from others. If someone notices the change you're embracing and compliments you on it, don't wave her kind words aside. Accept them. Say "thank you" with your shoulders back and head held high. You've earned it.

7. Pardon

Finally, women who are successful at choosing their habits know the power of pardon. So you didn't quite master your new habit today? Forgive yourself.

Your new habit isn't reaping the results you envisioned as quickly as you'd like? Forgive yourself.

You're consumed with regret that you didn't embrace this habit sooner? You're convinced you've wasted months or even years in which you could have been enjoying a better quality of life? Forgive yourself.

You took two steps forward — and thirteen steps back? Forgive yourself.

Pardon. Don't choose a new habit without it.

HABITUAL WINNERS

The habits we choose determine much of what we get out of life. Not everything, mind you, but enough that it's worth being intentional about which habits we embrace. I don't know what habits you need to choose to make peace with your body and with your thoughts and emotions about your body. I'm guessing, however, that even if you haven't identified all of them, you've got a pretty good idea where to begin.

So pick a healthy habit or two, then choose your perspective, prepare for success, interrupt the old habit when you need to, hang out with positive partners, be persistent, welcome pats on the back, and pardon yourself when you fail.

And if, after all that, you still end up at See's Candies or Bob's Big Boy, don't be too hard on yourself. Consider yourself in good company.

The woman standing in line in front of you is probably me.

GET A NEW BODITUDE

Questions for Personal Reflection or Group Discussion

• Sometimes all it takes is one or two good habits to lead the way, and soon other good habits fall into place. Think of two habits that, if you could embrace them, would make your life easier. Picture them, then say them out loud.

• What seems like it would be easier to do: *change* your habits or *choose* your habits? Why?

• If you are struggling to embrace a new habit, or regretting something you said or did in the past, how easy do you find it to forgive yourself for your blunders?

• Can you think of any habits that may be contributing to your funk about your body? If so, what are they?

- Have you considered giving up? Have you given up? If so, do you feel the freedom to get up tomorrow morning and gave it another shot?

8
CHOCOLATE IS
CHEAPER THAN THERAPY
MAKING PEACE WITH YOUR EMOTIONS

One Sunday morning I checked my e-mail and found a note from my daughter, just turned fourteen, who happened to be in Germany. She was backpacking around the countryside with her dad, and they had been there a week. With no cell phones or computers, and staying in a different hotel or youth hostel every night, communication had been limited to the few times they had wandered into an Internet café. So when I saw Kacie's name in my inbox, my heart jumped with joy! Unfortunately, I had an entirely different reaction when I read what she had to say:

Hi Mama,
    We are in Munich. I found the cutest little town ever! It's all old and it's from the Renaissance. I took tons of pictures. I can't wait to show you when I get home!!!

By the way, there is a chance I might have to stay here in Munich for another week. Dad is sick with some sort of throat infection, and he might need to go into a hospital. If that happens, I could probably stay by myself in a cheap hotel until he is better. There is a little market nearby, and I can get around the city on the trains, so please don't be scared, everything will be fine. Nothing to worry about.

Tonight we will stay in our regular hotel. Dad got some pills today, and if they make him better by tomorrow, he might not have to go to the hospital. I will send you a message when I know where I'll be. All is well and I miss you and love you a lot. ☺ Tell everybody I say hi.

Oh, gee, I might have been tempted to FREAK OUT if she hadn't added the comforting words "don't worry" or assured me she could take trains to get back and forth to the market from the CHEAP HOTEL ROOM she'd be living in by *herself* for a week!

I kicked into high gear, scouring the house for their travel itinerary and placing a dozen phone calls. I called a friend in the travel business. I called Kayla, my ex's current wife and Kacie's stepmom, and left an urgent message: Had she heard anything, or did she know how to reach them? Another friend helped me figure out how to get my expired passport renewed within twenty-four hours, then track down the number of the German hotel where Larry and Kacie were staying for one night before going their separate ways. Larry to hospital bed rest and my fourteen-year-old to a CHEAP HOTEL for a *week*.

When I finally reached Kacie and her dad by phone, there was good news. Whatever pills Larry took had kicked in. He was feeling better. There would be no hospital stay for him, nor a cheap hotel for my daughter. They were both doing fine, and their trip would continue as planned.

I, on the other hand, was probably going to need several bowls of ice cream and a three-pound bag of Fritos.

FEAR? SADNESS? ANGER? GRAB A SPOON

Stuff happens every day that freaks us out, doesn't it? Okay, maybe your barely-fourteen-year-old has never gotten almost stranded in Germany, but still . . . there are more than enough stressors and worries to go around for everyone.

It's a little foreign to me, but I'm realizing there is a segment of the human population that doesn't turn to food when they're upset. For years I didn't think such a creature existed. I thought people who get upset and don't eat were mythological beings, like werewolves or vampires or the tooth fairy. But the noneaters are real. I know, because I've met a few of them. Someone says, "I'm too upset! I can't eat a thing!" and I do a double take. I fight back the urge to hold up a mirror to see if they make a reflection. Who knows? Maybe vampires are real too.

But for me and many of my friends, intense emotions drive us to the pantry. Or the fridge. (Once I rescued a perfectly good half-eaten piece of chocolate cake from a waste basket, but that's just between you and me, okay?)

The good news is that using food to manage our emotions actually works, at least temporarily. The bad news is that it makes us feel bad about ourselves and our bodies, and *not* just temporarily. The good news is that we can learn new strategies to manage our emotions. The bad news is that it's not as easy as it sounds.

So let's go back to the part about how

intense emotions drive us to the pantry and see where we go from there. First, let's look at how we feel about our emotions. I have just recently become aware of how afraid I am of intense emotions. Not the intense happy ones, of course. I seek those out like size 9 pumps on a Manolo Blahnik clearance rack.

It's the *other* kind of emotions that I'm talking about.

I mentioned in an earlier chapter that I had been seeing someone I really liked. That was the good part. But after six months, there was just some stuff we couldn't resolve. So several weeks ago I did it. Hurt and upset about something that had happened, I ended things. This wasn't another one of those "we're *trying* to break up, but we can't stay away from each other" things. This time it was for real.

Before I got my car all the way out of his driveway, I was on my cell phone, calling a casual acquaintance and taking him up on his longstanding invitation to buy me a cup of coffee. I didn't want to date this man, and we both knew it. So what was I thinking?

Somewhere on the freeway en route to the downtown coffee shop where we planned to meet, it hit me hard. I wasn't thinking; I was reacting. I was so afraid of feeling sad over things not working out with you-know-who that I was propelling myself at seventy-five miles an hour into hanging out with someone I didn't really want to hang out with.

It dawned on me that, if I weren't speeding toward a distraction in the shape of someone buying me a cup of coffee, I'd be speeding toward something else. Like six tacos and a plate of cheesy nachos. Or two bowls of popcorn laced with Peanut M&M's. Something my body didn't need for fuel and that, at some level, I didn't even want to eat.

The point of this humiliating confession is that I'm realizing that, when I'm thrown off kilter, I'll do almost anything to regain emotional equilibrium. And my coffee date notwithstanding, most of the time when I'm terribly upset, my ballast of choice is food.

The image that comes to mind is a boat being tossed around in a choppy sea of circumstances. Living in dread of chaotic, uncomfortable emotions, I use food like sandbags to quickly counterbalance the impact of whatever rocks my world. When I'm hit with a wave of unexpected and unwanted emotions, the dilemma that seems to drive me is this: "If I don't use food as ballast, what then? What if I have all these strong emotions and the boat feels lopsided and it's uncomfortable and scary and I don't know what to do?"

I'm so afraid of intense negative emotions that I use food like a drug to calm myself down. Food can be used not only as emotional ballast but as a pretty effective tranquilizer too. In fact, emotional eating can even serve as a kind of self-hypnosis, sending us into a subtle trance.

Just this morning I woke up sad and worried, went to the kitchen to make coffee, and ended up, instead, sitting in an easy chair clutching a big bowl of popcorn left over from the night before. As I sat there methodically shoveling cold popcorn into my mouth and mulling over my problems, it dawned on me that my state of mind was detached and somewhat trancelike. Even my movements — the hypnotic hand-to-mouth thing I had going on — felt rhythmic and mesmerizing.

At that moment I wasn't zoning out on popcorn to escape my problems or even to try to balance my emotions, but to calm myself down enough so I could sit in the same room with my problems. In this food-induced trance, I was able to ponder things painful and horrible. They were things that, without the help of food, might have sent me running from the room.

Do you ever feel this way, as if some emotions are so unpleasant that they must be "snuck up on" while you're doing something else — like eating — which numbs your fear? As if the emotions are so intense, they are most safely viewed from a distance through a haze created by what and how we eat?

It makes me think of the mythological monster Medusa, who was so beautiful and terrifying with her hair of snakes that anyone who looked directly at her was immediately turned to stone. The man who finally slew her was able to get close enough to her only because he didn't look directly at her, but at her reflection in a mirrored shield.

Is this what emotional eating sometimes does for us? Allows us to interact with a dimmed and distorted image of our pain, so that we aren't completely undone by looking at it face to face?

EEK! IT'S AN EMOTION!

One night I wrote in my journal: "Why do my emotions scare me so much? That I can't just let them be? That I have to so quickly balance them out? Equalize them

116

with food? Neutralize them? It's like I'm terrified of hurt. Then again, maybe it's because sometimes the hurt takes me places that are scary. Places I'm not always sure I can find my way out of. Broken places that are dark and sad. And I don't always know how to stay out of those places except to avoid the emotions that lead me there."

Maybe you have felt some of these same things, or maybe you have different reasons for trying to tame your emotions with food. Maybe you were taught that intense emotions are wrong, or that "good girls" need to suppress their emotions so they can spend their energies taking care of other peoples' needs rather than their own. Perhaps you're afraid of feeling out of control.

I wish I knew ten easy steps to making peace with scary emotions. Or, hey, as long as we're dreaming, why not make it five easy steps? Better yet, how about a couple of quick thoughts and a magic pill?

I don't have any of those things. In fact, when it comes to this subject, some days I feel about as clueless as a box of hair. But here's what I do have — four strategies for taming scary emotions without resorting to misusing food or abusing our bodies.

The Mike-and-Sulley Strategy

Pixar's animated movie *Monsters, Inc.* tells the story of a little girl who befriends the scary monsters that inhabit her closet and the dark recesses beneath her bed. In developing a new perspective and relationship with her nemeses, she trades fear for freedom and life.

Why can't we do the same thing? Sometimes, when I find myself surrounded by big, hairy emotions that feel threatening or scary, I try to picture them looking a little like Sulley and Mike, the furry enemies-turned-BFFs who are the stars of the movie. The first couple of times I did this, it didn't help at all. The third time I tried it, the thought seemed so silly I actually cracked a smile. It hasn't revolutionized my life, but I think it has promise. I'll keep trying it and keep you posted. You try it too.

The Quantum-Leap Approach

I mentioned earlier that we often use food like ballast to regain emotional equilibrium when we feel rocked by adverse or unsettling circumstances. But there has to be a less-fattening way to balance our emotions.

Better yet, instead of balancing, what if we could transport ourselves into a better mood altogether? What if we could make the jump to a different place, not unlike Dr. Sam Beckett, the accidental time traveler? In the TV show *Quantum Leap,* which ran in the early 1990s, Scott Bakula played the time-warped quantum physicist who was involuntarily transported at the end of every episode into a different time period and even a completely different body.

I don't know about time periods or morphing bodies, but we all know there are things that transport us into different moods. Music, exercise, and laughter have this power. Sometimes a movie or book can transport us into a different emotional state. The next time you're struggling to stay away from the Doritos, turn on the Cartoon Network. Pop in a Bill Cosby DVD. Take a walk. Better yet, go to iTunes and download "Wild Thing," "Brick House," and "Bad to the Bone." Play it loud and get up and dance. Sing along. Make up motions to go along with the lyrics.

See what I mean? You feel better already.

The Six-Million-Dollar-Man Solution

In the 1970s, Lee Majors starred as astronaut Steve Austin in the TV series *The Six Million Dollar Man.* In the opening sequence to every episode, Steve is badly injured in a fiery lunar landing test. In a voiceover, as we see flashes of operating-room scenes, an authoritative voice tells us: "Gentlemen, we can rebuild him. We have the technology."

I love that line. "We have the technology."

There have been moments and seasons in my life when I came up against something that seemed hopeless. In those moments, I've been tempted to believe that whatever I was facing — problem, addiction, or emotion — was too big, too menacing, too permanent for me to handle. I can't tell you how often, in those times, I've quoted a paraphrased version of that goofy line from *The Six Million Dollar Man:* "We can fix this. We have the technology."

Just because I feel ill-equipped to handle something scary — like a big hairy emotion — doesn't mean that somebody, somewhere doesn't have the answer. *Somebody* has the technology.

A friend of mine admitted that, following a tough decade filled with stress and loss, he felt depleted of whatever internal resources he needed to cope with the emotions evoked by life's challenges. For the past six months, he's been working with a counselor to replenish his pool of coping skills. Learning how to stop thinking like a victim, how to be "present" in his current circumstances, and how to make healthier decisions regarding the future have vastly improved how he experiences and manages his emotions. This was the "technology" he needed to solve his inability to deal with them.

Reading books on codependency has helped me find healthy ways to address my need to save the world. Now, when I feel telltale emotions — like resentment, under-appreciation, that feeling of being "stretched too thin," or even a compassionate urgency to help others that leaves me feeling driven — I know what to do. Learning how to stop overmeeting the needs of others while un-dermeeting my own was the "technology" I needed to deal with some of my rogue emotions.

What technology is out there that can help you? Counseling? Prayer? Anger management classes? Grief workshops? Divorce-recovery classes? Find out, and then get the most from the best technology.

The Opie Connection

I love the scene, while opening credits roll, in *The Andy Griffith Show* where Andy and Opie are walking on a lakeside path, carrying fishing poles and holding hands.

When I take walks with my daughters, we look just like that. Except we don't carry fishing poles. And at fourteen and twenty-two, my girls are a lot taller than Ronnie Howard was at six. And, since growing my hair longer, strangers have finally stopped approaching me in grocery stores and confusing me with Ben Matlock. But other than that, the similarities are astounding.

Except I've noticed that Opie never gives Andy gum wrappers. When we walk, my girls are always trying to hand me gum wrappers. Or empty juice cartons. Or Popsicle sticks or *something.* They'll peel open a candy bar, then turn around and try to give me the wrapper. I'm always saying, "Do I look like a trash can to you?" and making them carry it in their own pockets until we find a real trash can.

I'm glad my heavenly Father doesn't say the same thing to me. Sometimes I find myself carrying something I don't want and don't know what to do with. There have been times when, weeping, I've barely managed to form the words, "God, I have no idea what to do with this. Can you please-pleaseplease carry this for a while?"

And the burden lifts. My circumstances and emotions might not have changed all that much. But something will have shifted. From me to God, I guess. And since he's walking beside me, it's not like my problems are all that far away. But at least they're not in my pocket anymore; they're in his. And sometimes, at that moment, that's all I need.

I don't know if it's a good sign that my "wisdom" on this subject is based on animated characters and sci-fi TV series. What I do know is that as we do these four things — devillainize our emotions, practice transitions from bad 'tudes to better moods, accept the belief that we can find and embrace the skills we lack, hold our God/Dad's hand as we walk and sometimes even ask him to carry burdensome debris — we may very well discover that food no longer has the hold on us it once did.

And best of all, we will have taken significant steps toward looking our most frighteningly intense emotions straight in the eye.

GET A NEW BODITUDE

Questions for Personal Reflection or Group Discussion

- What kinds of emotions feel too big for you to handle? Grief? Loss? Anger? Sadness? Others? What kinds of events have created these kinds of emotions for you?

- When you're faced with emotions that feel too threatening, what are some of the things you do to find relief? Which of these are healthy, and which are destructive?

- Do you think you have healthy skills and resources for dealing with painful emotions? What emotions do you handle well? What emotions don't you handle well?

9
DIEHARD CHOCOHOLICS ONLY GO TO RECOVERY MEETINGS FOR THE REFRESHMENTS

MAKING PEACE WITH YOUR ADDICTIONS TO FOOD

I've gotten addicted to the weirdest things. Watching *thirtysomething*. Painting wall trim. Humming "I'm a Little Teapot." And babies.

Every time I had a baby, I got addicted. I just couldn't get enough. The first time I got addicted was right after I'd given birth to Kaitlyn. The second time was eight years later, when I gave birth to Kacie. Junkies love company, and the second time there was another addict in the house. Kaitlyn and I would spend hours unable to tear our eyes away from the little mewing blond bundle who had recently inhabited our home and our hearts. Once, when Kacie was a little older, Kaitlyn observed in awe, "She has such a big personality for such a little body." We were addicted all right.

At one point I got addicted to garage sales. Eventually I honed my addiction to specific garage-sale finds, like floor lamps. I was addicted to floor lamps for several years. Now it's little printers for my computer. There must be seven little printers sitting around me in my office. Half of them even work.

I'm also addicted to grabbing a hammer and crowbar and taking down portions of walls in my home. The last time I did this, my friend Ashley and I were chatting in the family room when I looked at a wall and said, "That needs to go." We grabbed the appropriate tools and got to work. Everything was going perfectly until I started cutting out a wall stud and there was a flash and a pop and the house went dark. Six hundred dollars, one electrician, and two handymen later, the doorway I had envisioned turned out beautifully. Apparently, when it comes to a do-it-yourself project, two may be company, but five can get pretty darn expensive.

I've been addicted to in-home demolition since my first intoxicating foray into this rather unladylike hobby about three years ago. After being depressed for about six months while getting over my breakup with Skippy (read my book *Due to Rising Energy Costs, the Light at the End of the Tunnel Has Been Turned Off* for more of that story), I decided to throw a Halloween party to distract myself from my broken heart. Kacie, Kaitlyn, and I spent an entire month decorating every room in the house. We even decorated the ceilings.

But the crowning touch of our craziness occurred when I looked at a blank wall in my grand center hallway and said to Kacie, "Wouldn't it be cool to cut a huge, four-foot circle in the middle of that wall and decorate it like a monster mouth, and make people step through it to get into the room on the other side?"

Kacie, who was eleven at the time, said, "Sweet! Can we do it right now? Please, Mom, please? Can I get the hammer?"

I said, "Grab two hammers. And the Sawzall."

My niece, Gabriella, was there too, and the three of us hammered and sawed and squealed and laughed and coughed up drywall dust for hours. My sister Michelle snapped pictures. When Kaitlyn came home from college the following weekend, she walked in the front door, took one look at the huge monster mouth gracing the hallway, and said, "Yep. The jury's been out for years, but if they could see what I'm seeing right now, they'd come to a unanimous decision: you really are certifiably crazy."

People who came to our party were

amazed that I would go to that extreme measure. Sometimes, as they gawked admiringly, I confessed the truth, which was that I'd always wanted to put french doors in that spot, so our monster mouth wasn't as random as it seemed. It was really just phase one of a long-anticipated home-improvement project.

But I didn't.tell *everybody* the monster mouth was the first step in getting french doors installed. After all, why spoil a perfectly good reputation for being certifiably crazy?

YOU KNOW YOU'RE AN ADDICT WHEN . . .

You may have noticed that, in my list of personal addictions, I didn't mention food. This is because, despite the fact that many of us are proud owners of coffee mugs and T-shirts that say things like "I Heart Chocolate" and "Will Work for Cupcakes," it's just a joke, right? We love food, and we adore chocolate — and, sure, sometimes we can't stop eating to save our lives — but it's not a *real* addiction. And it's certainly not as dangerous as, say, my addiction to drywall demolition, right?

At least that's what I thought until I happened across the Web site of UCLA psychiatrist Dr. Roger Gould. I've tended to think of emotional eating as a compulsion. Gould uses the word *addiction*. I think his word is closer to the truth. After all, it's been said that you're addicted to something when you (a) have a hard time controlling how much you use of a particular substance, and (b) continue to use this substance regardless of negative consequences in your life.

According to Gould, the reason people like me (and maybe you) get addicted to food is because *it works:*

> It really is a powerful way to change the whole state of your mind, temporarily. If you are anxious, eating can rid you of anxiety. It can give you time to regroup. Some people have described how eating puts them into their own bubble, and makes all the worries go away for a while. Others have described a state of feeling insulated and protected instead of vulnerable and raw. When you are addicted, eating has become a way to silence your mind whenever it presents you with ideas or images you'd rather not deal with. In that sense, it does work; it temporarily banishes uncomfortable thoughts and the feelings associated with them. And when you are addicted to this

feeling, you have very little control over how much you eat.[1]

That certainly describes the role food can play in our lives. At least in my life. I'll be the first to admit that I'm addicted to the rush of disconnect, numbness, lethargy, and calm that follows an emotional-eating frenzy. And whenever I'm stressed or hurting, I crave that rush of numbness so strongly that I'm willing to sacrifice my health, my looks, my energy level, and even my feelings about myself to get it. And how different, really, is this from the experience of someone who is addicted to cigarettes, drugs, drinking, pornography, shopping, or gambling?

If you have done the yo-yo-dieting thing — unless you can look me square in the eye and tell me sincerely that you wanted to regain all that weight — it's possible that you're addicted too. The idea of emotional eating as an addiction isn't a completely new concept, but I have to admit it's one I've never explored before. But if emotional eating is an addiction, shouldn't the same recovery principles that apply to alcohol and drug addictions work for food as well?

It turns out that they do. Here are some nuggets of recovery wisdom that apply regardless of what we're addicted to.

HALT

Alcoholics Anonymous is credited with originating the acronym HALT, which stands for Hungry, Angry, Lonely, Tired. It is a quick assessment tool to help us recognize when we are most vulnerable to making a mistake or relapsing into an addiction. Feeling hungry, angry, lonely, or tired is very often the state we find ourselves in right before temptation strikes!

You may not be thinking about turning to food for comfort — yet — but you soon will be if you continue neglecting your legitimate needs. If you find yourself feeling hungry, angry, lonely, or tired, stop what you're doing and take care of business in a healthy way. Otherwise you may end up making a choice that you regret.

What's interesting is that I found this approach recommended on Web sites devoted to people who want to stop smoking, avoid mistakes in their careers, recover from addictions to drugs, or put a stop to emotional eating. I even read about it in an article telling poker players how to gamble better. According to the article, if you're in a high-stakes game and you find yourself feeling hungry, angry, lonely, or tired, you're at greater risk of making stupid mistakes.

What does this mean for you and me? When we find ourselves experiencing any of these four conditions, it's time to take action. Hungry? Eat something healthy. Angry? Pray about it, make a decision to let it go, forgive, take your anger out on a punching bag, see a counselor, or take a walk and cool off. If you're lonely, call someone, attend a worship service, or go hang out with friends. Tired? Have a banana and a cup of tea with honey, take a power nap, or even call it a day and go to bed.

TEMPTATION 911

Let's say you didn't HALT and now you can't get the thought of cheesecake a la mode out of your head. You're teetering on the verge of giving in to your food addiction. What can you do?

- Think ahead. It's easy to tell yourself this one cookie won't hurt, but be honest and think about how you're going to feel ten minutes from now when you've polished off the entire bag.
- Get outta Dodge. Leave the kitchen. Leave your house and go for a walk. Get in your car and get outta town if you have to. There's a story in the

Bible about a young man who ran screaming from the room to escape a seductress. Okay, I don't know if he was screaming. But he fled so quickly that he left his jacket behind. Maybe we should follow his example. Temptation is not always as tenacious as we think it is. Sometimes all it takes is a change of scenery to help us get a grip.

- Practice relaxation. When we're tense, we gravitate toward familiar patterns, even if they are destructive patterns. Being tense increases the urgency we feel to find relief wherever we can, even if it's at the bottom of a carton of ice cream. On the other hand, when we are relaxed, we are less driven. Less needy. We can think more clearly. We can make better decisions. Besides, you have to admit that even a hardcore chocolate craving would have to work hard to top a warm bubble bath in flickering candlelight amid the honeyed sounds of smooth jazz.

ENVISION A NEW LIFE

I like this nugget of wisdom from the Web site www.addictionsandrecovery.org, devoted to helping people recover from alcohol and drug addictions: "You don't recover from an addiction by stopping using. You recover by creating a new life where it is easier not to use."

What does this mean for you and me? It means that padlocking the pantry while we leave the rest of our lives unexamined and unaltered probably isn't going to work. Overcoming any addiction requires changes in paradigms and lifestyle. It requires new thoughts, new strategies, and new behaviors.

There is a saying in AA: nothing changes if nothing changes. When I read the following comment, also from the Web site www.addictionsandrecovery.org, it blew me away: "Recovery is difficult because you have to change your life, and all change is difficult, even good change. Recovery is rewarding because you get the chance to change your life. Most people sleepwalk through life. They don't think about who they are or what they want to be, and then one day they wake up and wonder why they aren't happy. If you use this opportunity for change, you'll look back and think of your addiction as one of the best things that ever happened to you."[2]

How amazing would *that* be? What if personal struggle turned into personal growth? What if my addiction became the catalyst for health and blessing in my life?

What if something that I'd been using for evil got turned around and was used for good instead?

THAT HIGHER-POWER THING

If any of the ideas in the previous paragraph sound familiar, maybe there's a reason. Maybe, like me, you've come across similar ideas expressed in the Bible. After all, Joseph said to his underhanded, conspiring siblings: "You intended to harm me, but God intended it for good to accomplish what is now being done, the saving of many lives" (Genesis 50:20).

In Romans 8:28 the apostle Paul assures us that if we love God and align ourselves with his plans for our lives, he can take everything we experience and use it for our good.

And King David wrote that God changed his sobbing into dancing, removed his mourning clothes, and dressed him in joy instead (see Psalm 30:11).

Indeed, the Bible is filled with stories that illustrate God's desire to turn chaos into order, weeping into joy, bondage into freedom, and shame into honor — which may be much of what AA's Higher Power thing is all about. After all, recovery groups dealing with everything from alcohol, sex, gambling, and food to shopping and smoking encourage participants to recognize that they are powerless to fix their problems by themselves and must turn to a Higher Power for help.

Whether you think you're a food addict or feel that you simply have a weakness, you are obviously seeking some change and better coping skills or you wouldn't have picked up this book. Are you trying to do it on your own? Or is there Someone omnipotent and wise you can turn to?

DROWNING IN A SEA OF EMOTIONS

Life can be turbulent, creating storms of raw emotions. Sometimes I feel like I'm drowning, and whether I binge eat for relief or simply cry myself to sleep, sometimes I wish I could trade all the unruly emotions for something sane and reliable. I need something I can really use, something that doesn't generate much drama. Like maybe a toaster oven or a sturdy extension cord. But, alas, in my life and perhaps in your life, too, there will always be seasons when dark skies descend and volatile waves rise and our worlds get slapped around.

A long time ago a small band of men found themselves in circumstances just like this. Far out on a lake in the middle of the night, buffeted by wind and waves, these seasoned fishermen were anxious and afraid. Then they saw something that must have *really* made their hairs stand on end: a man they didn't recognize in the gloom was walking toward them across the surface of the storm-tossed waters. When the man was close enough, he yelled through the wind, "Take courage! It's me! Don't be afraid!"

It was their Teacher, the man they called Lord, the man who said he was the Son of God. At that moment Peter — dear impetuous Peter — hollered back at the "apparition" who seemed undaunted by the churning waters. "If it's really you, Lord, tell me to walk across the water to you!"

Jesus must have smiled at that, but since it was dark, I guess we'll never know for sure. What we do know is that he issued an invitation, "C'mon then!" and Peter swung one leg and then the other over the splintery side of the dizzily rocking boat.

Can you imagine how disorienting that would be, to thrust your feet where there is nothing solid and expect to stand? Surprisingly, stand he did, and then he took a step, and then another, and another still. Suddenly Peter was doing the impossible, something he'd never seen done before except by one man, the Man/God standing with him in the storm. For several exhilarating moments, Peter was walking tall on top of churning waves. What a thrill that must have been!

Then fear took over, and suddenly he was sinking up to his ankles, then his knees, then his waist, in choppy, angry water. Still sinking, he cried out, "Lord! Save me!"

And Jesus reached out and caught him.[3]

What a trip! I'll bet you a shekel to a donut that if someone offered Peter the chance to go back in time and undo anything about that night, he'd say "No way!" I don't think he would change a thing: not the anxiety he felt as the storm began to gather, not the fear he felt while being buffeted by the wind and waves, not his confusion when he spotted a lone figure approaching across the water, not the excitement and terror he must have felt as Jesus hollered back, "C'mon then! Come to me across the stormy waters!" Peter wouldn't change the rush of adrenalin as he swung his legs over the side of the boat and lowered himself onto the churning water, the surreal exhilaration of walking on the water, the shame of failure as he started to sink, or the panic he must have felt as the deep threatened to consume him. And he especially wouldn't change the indescribable relief and awe he must have felt as Jesus pulled him out of the hungry waves.

If you ask me, fear and panic and even shame seem like small prices to pay in exchange for the chance to experience such a thrilling and miraculous intervention! And was there anything that Jesus did for Peter that was less than extraordinary? When he invited Peter to come to him across stormy waters, was that not amazing? When he empowered Peter to rise above his circumstances, was that not miraculous? And when Jesus snatched Peter to safety, was that not a moment rich and sacred?

Looking at Peter's life, it's easy to see how he might welcome a thousand storms if even one of them allowed him to experience Jesus in the way he experienced him that night. But what about my storms? And what about yours? Is it possible the storms offer us the chance to experience something miraculous, amazing, rich, and sacred?

I was talking to my daughter Kaitlyn about the ideas in this chapter when she said, "I've read something about that!" She told me about a book in which the author talked about his conversations with numerous people who had been persecuted for their faith in God. The author was amazed that on more than one occasion, his subjects began to weep, admitting there was one thing they desperately missed from their season of persecution. There was one thing they longed to recapture and never could. They missed experiencing Jesus now as they had during those desperate times.

Then Kaitlyn grew thoughtful and added, "I can understand that feeling. Sometimes I miss how close I felt to the Lord during my freshman year of college. I think I was still reeling from your and dad's divorce, John and I had just broken up, one of my roommates and I were at each other's throats, you and I had been fighting about stuff, Dad was talking about looking for a job in another state . . . All that to say, I was a mess!

"And I remember one day walking through the supermarket. I wasn't pushing a cart — I think I was just there for a couple of things — and I was walking through the juice aisle when I just couldn't take one more step. I fell down, on my knees, my face near the linoleum, and I was sobbing and sobbing. I started praying, but I wasn't asking the Lord for a miracle or anything big or important; I was just asking him to pleasepleaseplease help me get to my feet and get back to my car. I was that desperate. I needed him that bad for something that basic. 'Just help me get off this floor.' "

She added, "Sometimes I think when we're really desperate, when we have no place else to turn, we really do get to experience Jesus in ways we don't when everything is great or even tolerable in our lives."

I don't know what storms you're facing or what obstacles are making you feel overwhelmed, but can I make a suggestion? The next time you're buffeted by life and your emotions roil up huge and threatening as a result, instead of trying to dull or appease those scary emotions with food, try this. I promise I'll try it, too. Look out across your stormy sea of circumstances. Then squint your eyes against the driving wind, and try to peer past all the crashing waves of emotions. What do you see? Could it be that Someone is drawing close and calling to you through the chaos? That he is hollering out an invitation? Beckoning you to climb out of your splintery, rickety safety zone (believe me, it's not all that safe anyway!), and come to him?

Say yes. Step out of the boat. I know the waves are scary; they scare me, too! And even though huddling blindly in the hull of the boat may seem like the best available option, it's not. Especially not when there's a Man/God standing with us in the storm with his hands extended, inviting us to stop using our addictions to avoid the waves — and asking us to come to him instead.

And if we accept his invitation, what then? Will he miraculously empower us to rise above it all? Or will we still find ourselves in some dark and scary places from which he will eventually rescue us? I think the answer to both questions is yes.

The bad news is that storms are scary. The good news is that the Lord of the waves and the Master of winds says, "Come."

GET A NEW BODITUDE

Questions for Personal Reflection or Group Discussion

Addiction is a hard word to use, especially in regard to any of your own habits. Who wants to admit that their tendency to rely on a substance — even if it's only food — to face difficult issues in life might be an addiction? Ask yourself these questions to help you think through what you turn to when life feels overwhelming.

- Do you use food to cope? Could you be addicted to the rush of relief that food can provide?

• Do you have a hard time controlling what you eat? Do you continue to abuse food regardless of the negative consequences in your life?

You don't have to be in the middle of an emotional storm to say yes to Jesus. You don't even have to put this book down. Just say yes, right now, where you are. Your prayer can be as simple as this: *Jesus, I don't understand exactly how this all works, but Karen's telling me that you're the Son of God, that you're reaching for me, that you love me, that you want to empower and rescue me, that you want to intervene in my life in ways rich and sacred. It goes against reason, and it might even go against how I've been taught, but she's about as transparent as they come and, you know what, I'm going to believe her. So my answer is yes. Please begin to show me in the coming hours and days what that means. I'm climbing out of the boat and trusting you with my heart, my life, my soul. Save me, Lord. Make me your own.*

10

IF BEAUTY IS MORE THAN SKIN DEEP, WHY DON'T WE HAVE MAKEUP FOR INTERNAL ORGANS?

MAKING PEACE WITH YOUR IDEA OF WHAT IS BEAUTIFUL

Last week I got a free makeover at a department store, and with several years of therapy, I should recover completely from the experience.

It started out fine. As the makeup consultant ran cool fingers over my cheekbones, she commented to her assistant, "She has nice bone structure." I hid a small smile. This was, after all, the very reason I'd agreed to a makeover in the first place! It had been a stressful week, and I needed a lift. A few compliments from a commission-hungry saleswoman were just what the doctor ordered.

The consultant cleansed my face with Rejuvenating Foaming Cleanser. She toned it with Age-Defying Toning Lotion. She moisturized it with Dew of Youth Revitalizing Face Silk.

Suddenly she froze, her hand inches from my face. She peered closer at the skin beneath my eyes. Then she clucked her tongue and shook her head. She nudged her assistant and said, "Flakes."

Her assistant sadly agreed: "Cheap mascara."

The consultant turned to me. "What brand of mascara do you use?"

I told her. The two women rolled their eyes. "That explains it," said one. "No wonder," said the other.

"It's hardly cheap," I protested. "It costs fifteen dollars a tube."

The consultant cleared her throat, then paused a beat. "Ours costs forty-eight."

I set my jaw. "I love this mascara," I said. The last time I remembered speaking with this tone, I was four years old and stomping my foot.

The consultant fumbled under the counter and found a bottle of some sort of solvent. I think it was turpentine. She sloshed some on a cotton ball and said, "I'll get off what I can, but you may want to consider having your lashes surgically replaced."

Her assistant nodded. "Or sandblasted."

The consultant swabbed at my eyes. She applied foundation to my face. She highlighted my cheek bones with blush. She said, "Now I'm going to apply a few dabs of Age-Erasing Line Abolisher to the area around your eyes. Dabbing with my fourth finger, of course, because it applies the least pressure to fragile skin. This product will do wonders for your wrinkles."

She dabbed — gently so as not to inflict any more damage to my apparently time-weathered face — then turned to her assistant. "Makes a world of difference, doesn't it?"

Her assistant gawked. "Amazing. It takes ten years off her face."

The consultant nodded. "She could pass for fifty now, don't you think?"

I said, "I'm forty-eight."

The assistant whispered to me, "Plastic surgery costs thousands of dollars. This little bottle costs less than two hundred."

The consultant announced, "And now for the finishing touch . . ." Brandishing a tube of mascara, she wiped the wand across my lashes several times, then stopped and pouted. "I'm afraid it's not going to look right, not with the residue from that *other* brand."

Her assistant patted her arm and said soothingly, "It's not you. You've done wonders. She looks so much better than before."

Hoping to change the subject, I gestured

146

to a framed portrait of a young woman. "Is that a relative?" I was guessing niece.

The consultant said, "That's my grand-daughter."

It was my turn to gawk. "Granddaughter? You don't look old enough to be her mother."

"Thank you. I'm very careful with my skin regimen."

"I guess so."

"Imagine how youthful you'd look if you'd started using our products fifteen years ago."

Her assistant said, "There's always dam-age control."

The consultant brightened. "Of course there is. Hand her the list, will you?"

The assistant handed me a price list of the various products that were, at that moment, engaged in damage control on my face. I looked at the total and said, "I'll come back when I win the lottery."

I tossed the list in the trash on my way to the car. After all, if I were going to spend that kind of money, I'd put one of my kids through medical school. Or maybe help one of them get a doctorate in psychology. I figure a few more makeovers like this one and I'll be grateful to have a therapist in the family.

Hey, Gorgeous!

What's beautiful to you?

When I was dating the guy I mentioned back in chapter 8, he told me he'd watched a documentary on beauty and apparently, when it comes to facial features, there's some sort of mathematical ratio that is considered "classically beautiful" in most cultures. We measured my face. He said my brows were a little close. I said no problem, tomorrow morning when I draw them on I'll leave more space between them.

I love makeup. I love makeup because I enjoy how I look and feel when I wear it. It's also fun to apply, kind of like a grownup version of a coloring book. I like makeup so much that I had my eyebrows tattooed and I still apply eyebrow pencil, although I'll admit I'm leaving a little more space between them these days.

I've never balanced a checkbook in my life and my 401(k) is trashed, but thank God my facial-features ratio is balanced and intact.

I don't know what Karen Kartes thinks about classical facial ratios, but I had a chance to interview this effervescent thirty-nine-year-old woman about her definition of beauty.[1] And what struck me is how powerfully her definition of beauty defined her life for more than twenty years.

"My mom has seven sisters, all with voluptuous bodies," she told me. "When I was sixteen, I remember looking at the women in my family and seeing what I would be inheriting as I grew older. At the same time, I was bombarded with images from society that told me 'beautiful' needed to look like something else. I remember looking at my family and thinking, *That's not what I want. I'm going to look different than that.*"

Karen began running at age fifteen, not because she enjoyed the sport, but because she believed that the more calories she burned, the more she could control her size and shape. Then, in her twenties, Karen took a public-relations position with a fitness-equipment manufacturer. She often attended industry events where, she noticed, "everyone was uber fit." Concluding that "fitting in" meant wearing a size 2 or 3, she became further obsessed with using exercise to control her body.

About that time, she became engaged to a man who was later diagnosed with a chronic illness and died two years later. Karen remembers, "Between the stress of that experience — and the obsessions I had bought into — I was definitely depriving myself of nutrition. I was eating, at most, a salad a day for strength and purging anything else, throwing it up to get it out of my body. I've read about eating disorders and, yes, it's about controlling your life, and, yes, it's about pressure from society and body types, but it goes deeper than that. When life feels unpredictable or chaotic and you realize there's one thing you can control — even at the price of your own health — you hang onto that."

In her thirties, Karen began working for World Vision, a faith-based nonprofit hunger-relief organization. The shift from a corporate environment to nonprofit put Karen in, as she describes it, a "happier place." She says, "I loved my job. My life felt more stable. I began to see the error of my ways."

She also began to see life from a broader perspective. She says World Vision's global focus made her more aware of health and living conditions in other countries. Realizing there are people who are eating one meal a day — not because that's what they want to do, but because they don't have a choice — was sobering.

Karen's personal demons quieted for a season; she began running marathons again — this time to raise money for charity. Or so she thought. Before long, old patterns had reemerged. Even though she was no longer binging and purging, Karen became obsessed with restricting calories. Eventually whittling herself down to a size 3, she says, gave her an ecstatic feeling. She told herself, "Wow! Look! I've defied my family genetics! I'm not pear shaped! I'm a stick, and I like it!" Today she adds, "It's true, you look in the mirror, and you can't see reality. Looking back, I know now I wasn't in a healthy place."

And she wasn't. Two years ago, Karen crashed and burned. Years of abusing her body and depriving herself of nutrition finally caught up with her. "I didn't have motivation to go on," she explains. "I felt bad about myself and where I'd ended up. I was having flashbacks of traumatic times in my life. It was very scary. It felt like someone was after my soul, and it wasn't God. I didn't make any plans to hurt myself, but I remember going to sleep thinking, *If I don't wake up, that's okay with me.*"

DO YOU THINK YOU'RE BEAUTIFUL?

Do you think you're beautiful? On the surface, it's a pretty simple question. And yet the answer can change daily. When I ask myself that question, sometimes my answer is yes. Sometimes it is no. Sometimes I throw in an explanation or condition, like "I would be beautiful if . . ." or "I'm only beautiful when . . ."

What about you? Do you think you're beautiful?

And if we don't think we're beautiful — or if we don't think we're beautiful enough — what then? To what lengths are we willing to go to feel beautiful?

Apparently I'm willing to go the length of a good eyelash extension. I say this because last year Skippy — a former love interest now living out of state — was flying into town on business, and we made plans to meet for dinner. (Of course, his name isn't really Skippy, but you'll have to read *Due to Rising Energy Costs, the Light at the End of the Tunnel Has Been Turned Off* to find out more). Anyway, a week before seeing him, I was so worried about the twenty pounds I'd gained that I paid one hundred fifty dollars to get eyelash extensions, because, as we all know, if you've got great lashes a man won't notice that you're fat.

I'm sad to say that Skippy's plans changed and we didn't get to see each other after all. But I did get beautiful lashes out of the deal.

I've met drop-dead-gorgeous women who are ashamed — not just embarrassed but ashamed — of some feature of their bodies that doesn't fit the cookie-cutter beauty mold. One stunning blonde I know says she can't stand the length of her waist. I know petite women who are humiliated over their B-cup breasts, and buxom women who would give, if not their right arm, at least a good twenty pounds from their abdomens or thighs if they could experience a single day as a size 3.

Sometimes the urge to feel beautiful goes beyond longing and wishful thinking. Sometimes it can lead us down dark paths that — as soon as we've left the city lights far behind us and it's too late to turn around — fill us with dread and make us wonder why we ever left home at all.

TURNING POINT

Realizing she was in crisis, Karen Kartes took a leave of absence from her job to spend time with her family, seek professional help, and try to figure out what had gone so horribly wrong. She says she'll never forget the terrible day her parents came to help her pack so she could move back home with them. "It was a few weeks before my thirty-eighth birthday, and I couldn't function. I was depressed and scared where my mind was going. My parents were wonderful and accepting, but it was awful. I remember riding in the back seat of their car, feeling like a child."

Karen, raised Catholic, says she never stopped believing in God even though in her twenties she'd taken a hiatus from living as if she did. During her engagement, when her fiancé became a believer in Jesus Christ, Karen took a second look at her relationship with God. She began attending church again and felt closer to God than she had in a long time, but she also felt haunted by the thought that she needed to somehow earn his love. "I've always had perfectionist tendencies," she says, "so I figured if anyone could earn God's love, it was going to be me. Here I was, working for a nonprofit, doing good things in the world, working hard to keep my body under control. There was a certain amount of pride and vanity in all that, but it was also rooted in perfectionism."

So when her world fell apart, she found herself back in her parents' home. She was malnourished, depressed, unable to think clearly, and in an outpatient recovery program. No wonder she felt abandoned by the God she had tried so hard to please. And yet . . . it was in that dark place that God began to speak to her. "In the depths of my depression I felt God whispering to me. I felt him saying, 'You know all these people around you? These people telling you that you haven't been living in a healthy way? Listen to them. I've put them here to take care of you. I want you well.' "

Karen adds, "As I started healing and thinking more clearly, I felt God telling me he created me the way I am for a reason. I needed to embrace who I was and stop trying to control my life and my body in ways that were, in reality, killing me."

Now, two years later, Karen says she's in a good place physically, emotionally, and spiritually. She also admits that changing her thinking — while worth the effort — has not always felt comfortable. "Today I'm a size 8 which — for me and my family genetics — is a really healthy place to be. I'm thinking more clearly. But as I was gaining weight and becoming healthier — I won't kid you — it was hard going through my closet, pulling stuff out and thinking, *Will I ever wear this again?* Sometimes even now I'll see a picture of myself from the old days and think, *Wow! I was really cut back then . . .* But then I remind myself what it cost me. If it's a choice between being stick thin or being healthy and mentally alert, there's no contest. I still exercise, but I don't push myself. I love the endorphin rush and sense of well-being, but I no longer use it as a form of control. Instead, I see it as something I do for heath and well-being and for fun. I'm really content."

Fascinated with the idea of merging her professional and personal experiences, Karen says, "I know that my depression came out of depriving my body of essential nutrients, which affected my brain health. One of the things I'm really interested in right now is how nutrition impacts mental health in developing nations."

The other thing that has changed for Karen is her definition of beauty. "I come from a long line of pear-shaped women," she laughs. "This used to be a source of shame for me; now it's a source of pride. It's beautiful to me now. I think it's wonderful and beautiful to be a fuller body type if that's what you've been given."

I asked her how she managed to broaden her definition of beauty.

"Being exposed to other cultures through my work has definitely helped," she said. "The more I travel, the more I realize that many sizes and shapes are beautiful. And then I've changed. Sometimes I wish I could go back and redo those lost years. The depression, in particular, was especially debilitating. I never want to live through that kind of hell again. But I wouldn't trade the lessons I've learned for anything. I know now that God didn't abandon me and that he allowed me to go through that valley so I could get the help I needed and get healthy. I'm more passionate than ever about helping others so they don't fall into the same pit. And I finally realize that God accepts me, and that's a beautiful thing."

IS YOUR IDEA OF BEAUTIFUL TOO NARROW?

Can a pear-shaped body be beautiful? What about a wider-than-average smile? Can crooked teeth fit inside the box labeled "beautiful"? How about freckles? Or love handles?

How about a midlife body? I mean, let's be real. The last time I had perky breasts I was at Knott's Berry Farm, free-falling 120 miles an hour on a ride called the Parachute Drop. Can I still be beautiful?

How do we broaden the repertoire of shapes and images we find beautiful?

I'm still working on this one myself. For starters, you and I could follow the example of Anne whose strategy, described in chapter 2, involved finding pictures of "real" women in every size and shape and taping the images to her fridge and mirrors.

We could follow in the footsteps of Kaitlyn, who transformed her idea of beautiful by standing naked in front of a mirror and speaking truth over her body.

Like Karen Kartes, we could travel abroad, expanding our boundaries and, in the process, falling in love with the beauty inherent in diversity.

We can also tell the critical voices in our heads to shut up, and in their place we can start listening for the still, small voice of our Creator as he whispers to us. And, just like Karen, this is what we will hear him say:

Guess what? I knew exactly what I was doing when I made you. You are wonderfully made. I know you, inside and out. In fact, I knew you when you were still in your mother's womb and I've loved you from the very beginning. If you could see my face, if you could see my eyes and how I'm looking at you with such love and delight right now, you'd see yourself differently too. You'd begin to realize how beautiful and precious you really are.

The truth is that your beauty and worth aren't tarnished because a fickle society gets a whim, or because your parents made mistakes, or because someone didn't love you the way he should have. None of those people or circumstances made you beautiful or precious, so they can't unmake your beauty or your worth. The truth is that your beauty and worth are bestowed by me, redeemed through me, and revealed in me. And I would give my life for the chance to, every day of your life and on into eternity, show you and tell you truths about your beauty, worth, purpose, and destiny.

How I long to show you what I see when I look at you! You'll never see it in a mirror, or even in the eyes of a parent. Or find it in the embrace of a lover. Oh, you may catch glimpses there, but those glimpses will be distorted and fleeting and will only leave you yearning and desperately searching for the next illusive glimpse, and the one after that, and the one after that.

It's as if you're scraping your knees in the dirt, peering through tiny cracks and peepholes in the fence, while I'm standing here wanting to give you the keys to the garden gate and walk with you through the glorious landscape that is you. I created this garden, with great love and according to a plan. And if it's being held hostage by weeds and disarray, I can redeem it. And as you and I cultivate and explore it together, you're going to be amazed — you really are! There is beauty and magic in this place. And intention. And design. And treasure! And I haven't even begun to share with you all my wonderful plans for your future!

But I can't show you who you are while your eyes are glued to the mirror. Everything you long to see, I long to reveal to you. You are beautiful. You are loved. There is mystery and purpose in your design. Will you let me show you?

GET A NEW BODITUDE

Questions for Personal Reflection or Group Discussion
- Do you think you are beautiful? List the reasons you think you are beautiful. Or, if you said no, what are the reasons you feel that you're not?

- What are the factors that helped define

---

what you think is beautiful and what is not? The media? Your parents? Your friends? Men in your life? The Internet? Past circumstances?

- What is more important to you, health or beauty? To what length are you willing to go to feel beautiful by today's standards? What is the craziest thing you've done for the sake of perceived beauty?

- What do you think of the idea that it is only through a relationship with our Creator that you and I can gain a clearer picture and deeper understanding of our beauty and worth?

11

Burn Calories While You Sleep Without Strapping Yourself to a Treadmill

MAKING PEACE WITH YOUR METABOLISM

One morning at nine on the dot I heard a series of piercing whistle blasts coming from my front porch. I opened the door and found Joe, with a whistle in his mouth and wearing workout shorts, army boots, and a black T-shirt with SERGEANT printed boldly across the front.

Well, that's one way to start the morning.

Five minutes later we were in the middle of warm-up stretches when I heard shuffling and glanced toward the living-room doorway. There stood Kaitlyn and Kacie and a couple of their friends, having just tumbled out of beds and wearing an array of pajamas, T-shirts, and sweats. Home on summer vacation, the girls had been sleeping upstairs, their open bedroom windows directly above the front porch.

Kacie turned a sleepy face to the other girls and explained, "Oh. That's Joe. He makes Mom work out."

Kaitlyn yawned and said, "Wow! Cool. You go, Mom!"

Kacie added, "Yeah we're proud of you, Mom."

Joe said, "Good morning, girls! Now that you're awake, I have resistance bands for each of you."

I brightened at the thought. "Join us!"

All four girls turned back toward the hallway stairs.

"Hey!" I said. "Where are you going?"

Kaitlyn said, "Back to bed."

Kacie added, "Yeah. We said we were *proud* of you, Mom. We didn't say we were *insane* like you. G'night."

Joe and I worked out for forty minutes. My least-favorite exercise was the one using the sliders. With my palms on the floor and my body crouched in some sort of runners-starting-block stance with plastic sliders beneath my feet, I was supposed to pump my legs like I was running. Or climbing. In fact, Joe called this particular torture routine the Mountain Climber.

As soon as he barked out the order, I muttered, "We live in Colorado Springs. If I wanted to climb a fourteener, I'd just drive over to Pikes Peak."

Joe said, "By the time I'm through with you, you'll be sprinting the Peak."

I don't think he was joking.

METABOLISM: THE MAGIC VARIABLE

One afternoon Joe tried to explain the math part of losing weight. Apparently it's all about using up more calories than you take in, or something like that. Anyway, he was talking about how, if you use up thirty-five hundred more calories than you take in, you lose a pound.

"That's the part I never understand," I said. "It sounds like a cut-and-dried formula, but isn't there a variable? Don't people with a fast metabolism burn calories faster, while those with a slow metabolism take longer to lose weight?" And then, the obvious question: "What is metabolism anyway, and how do I speed mine up?"

Turns out *metabolism* is the word for the collection of chemical reactions that enables our bodies to take the energy in food — which is measured in calories — and break it down into energy our cells can use. Metabolism also determines when and how our cells use this fuel and — here's the rub — whether we stockpile the extra fuel we don't need as muscle (good) or as body fat (less good).

If you ask me, I don't want something with that much say-so working against me;

I want it working *for* me. Instead of burning calories slowly and storing extra fuel as body fat when I eat more than I need, I want my metabolism working hard to burn up all the calories I eat, *plus* burn up some extra fat. And when I do take in more calories than I need, I want my metabolism to *stop* storing it as fat and start stockpiling it as muscle.

Of course I also want a million dollars and a date with Jack Black. So am I reaching for the moon or do I have a chance? (At revamping my metabolism, I mean. I'm starting to lose hope about Jack.)

GEE THANKS, MOM AND DAD

The bad news is that our metabolisms are, in part, determined by our DNA, meaning there are factors we can't change. But whether our parents gifted us with a tortoise's metabolism or a hare's, I figure it's better than the alternative — no metabolism. This is because metabolism equals life. Anything organic — people, plants, animals, even refrigerator mold — metabolizes energy and, as a result, lives and grows.

Whether we train our metabolisms to help us grow wisely — or just wider — is up to us. Even though we can't control our DNA, there are five things we can do to take whatever we've been given and get it working for us rather than against us.

1. Wake Up Your Metabolism with Muscle!

Joe's first piece of advice was simply this: "The most important key to revving up your metabolism is muscle." As he explains it, the simple act of moving my body as I work out with weights temporarily revs up my metabolism and burns calories. But there's a second benefit to building muscle that lasts long past the actual workout.

The more muscle I have, the more calories my body burns even when resting or sleeping. This is called my basal — or resting — metabolic rate. If I were a car, this is how much gas I would burn while idling in the driveway. Now, when it comes to my car, naturally I don't want to use up a lot of gas just sitting. But when it comes to my body using up calories while I'm watching television or sleeping, that's another story! Burn, baby, burn!

2. Remember That Cardio Is King

Cardiovascular exercise is another metabolism booster. Cardiovascular exercises include jogging, biking, swimming, fast walking, jumping rope — you know, all the stuff that leaves you slightly breathless.

(Notice I didn't include as a cardio activity "watching any movie starring Keanu Reeves." I left this out for two reasons: First, I'm still hoping for that call from Jack Black before I move onto Keanu. And second, I'm not a personal trainer or anything, but I'm pretty sure the breathlessness is supposed to come from exercise.)

Just like with weight training, the simple act of moving your body as you work out will rev up your metabolism and burn calories. Also like weight training, cardio delivers a second benefit that lasts longer than the actual workout. This is because high-intensity cardio creates an oxygen debt in your body, meaning your body is recovering and therefore operating at a higher metabolism — and burning extra calories! — hours after you leave the gym. In other words, exercise in the morning and you'll enjoy the benefits of a souped-up metabolism all day long!

3. Take Ordinary Opportunities to Move Your Body

Any extra movement throughout your day boosts your metabolism. Magazine articles have been addressing this for years. People are always telling us to increase our activity by parking at the far end of every parking lot, taking stairs instead of elevators, hand delivering interoffice messages instead of e-mailing them, wearing a pedometer and trying to log five thousand or more steps throughout the day.

These are all good suggestions, but here's something you may not have read before: Joe suggests something he calls the Commercial Olympics. Since most of us watch two to four hours of television a day (and remain stationary during commercials), using commercial breaks to get in shape can be a good use of otherwise wasted time. During one commercial do lunges. During the next commercial do push-ups. During a third commercial do crunches, squats, or jog in place.

During the next set of commercials, dive into three or four minutes of power house-cleaning. Run a load of laundry to the washer. Vacuum just one room. See how many dishes you can do before your program starts again. Take your dog for a three-minute jog up and down your street. Clean all your bathroom mirrors. You'd be surprised at what you can accomplish — and how many calories you can burn — in three minutes.

4. Eat Stuff That Takes More Calories to Process

Get more mileage from your metabolism by eating foods that take more energy to process. Whole foods — meaning foods that are unprocessed or unrefined — are harder for your body to break down. To extract fiber and nutrients from whole foods, your body has to take chains of molecules and break them down into smaller versions so they can be absorbed into your bloodstream. This all takes energy, aka calories. Processed foods are much easier to digest, taking less work, meaning fewer calories are required.

5. Eat Smaller Meals More Often

Eating triggers digestion, which requires calories. So even if you decide to have a Quarter Pounder with supersize fries, if you divide it into six parts and eat it at intervals throughout the day — triggering your digestion six times instead of just once — you'll burn more calories.

So there you have it. To get every bit of mileage from your metabolism that you can, try these five things: build more muscle, get more cardio exercise, find even small ways to move more throughout the day, eat whole foods, and eat smaller meals more often.

Just don't tell Joe that I suggested a supersize order of fries. He could assign me an extra set of Mountain Climbers for that comment.

GET A NEW BODITUDE

Questions for Personal Reflection or Group Discussion
- Are you pretty active, or are you more of a couch or office potato? Rate your activity level on a scale of one to ten. Are you satisfied with how much activity your body gets throughout the day?

- What would it take to get you moving? We talked about three kinds of activity — weight training, cardiovascular exercise (biking, stair climbing, fast walking, jogging or running, swimming, and so forth), and finding small ways to get off your duff and move a little more. If you were going to incorporate one of these three things into your life, which would it be?

- Tell me your thoughts on processed foods compared to whole foods. We're talking apple juice versus eating a raw apple, instant mashed potatoes versus a baked potato (including the skin), cheese puffs versus carrots, white bread versus brown rice, Twinkies versus . . . oh, I don't know . . . maybe bell peppers. (Okay, so maybe that last one wasn't the best comparison, but you get the idea.) On a scale of one to ten — one being Fast Food Queen and ten being Euell Gibbons who is famous for his quirky line, "Ever eat a pine tree? Some parts are edible" — where are you? Where would you like to be?

12

WHY CAN'T THE WITNESS-PROTECTION PROGRAM HIDE ME FROM MOTHER NATURE AND FATHER TIME?

MAKING PEACE WITH YOUR BODY

Once upon a time there was a chaste and beautiful princess who married a handsome prince with thoughts of a very sexy, happily-ever-after life floating in her head like puffs of dandelion seeds. Unfortunately her honeymoon didn't exactly go as planned. Neither did the first months of her marriage. She bought lingerie. She lit candles. She suggested taking steamy showers together. When none of that worked, she came home with a highly romantic movie and edible panties. Nothing she did seemed to change things.

One day she looked in the mirror. She breathed into her hand to check her breath. She patted the corners of her eyes looking in vain for wrinkles. She even spun around and evaluated her bottom, which was a perfectly fine bottom as far as bottoms go. She was all of twenty-one, with a cute figure, no cellulite, and perky breasts. Her mirror nodded, gave an uh-huh and three snaps, and said, "Girl, you got it goin' on."

The princess's eyes filled with tears. Speaking to her reflection, she whispered the terrible question that gnawed at her soul: "But mirror, mirror on the wall, why am I the least desired of all?"

The mirror had no answer.

Confused, lonely, and rejected, the princess sought comfort in food. When that helped a little, she spooned up more comfort. Pretty soon she was eating three square meals of comfort plus as many consoling snacks as she could reasonably fit into a day. (At times, junk food even appeared in her dreams. But since dreams are calorie free, for the purposes of this story we're going to let it slide.)

Several years later she was busy doing something — probably eating — when she was caught off guard by her reflection in a mirrored closet door. She stood and took a long look. She checked her breath. It smelled like cookies. She looked for wrinkles, but the weight in her face filled them out nicely. She turned sideways and studied her bottom, which was much larger than it had ever been before.

The mirror pursed its lips and looked away.

The princess said sadly, "Mirror, mirror on my door . . . don't worry, it's all right. I don't ask that question anymore."

WHAT PROBLEMS ARE YOU SOLVING WITH THE SIZE OF YOUR BODY?

Earlier you and I talked about the relationship between our emotions and food and how — when we feel overwhelmed with emotions we can't handle — it's tempting to use food as ballast to balance things out. Likewise, when we feel overwhelmed with circumstances we don't know how to handle or problems we're not sure how to solve, it's tempting to use the size of our bodies as ballast. Some boats are equipped with pumps that can balance and stabilize the boat by pumping water into spaces on one side of the craft, to restore stability in rough seas. People aren't that different. We often do the same thing when our worlds get rocked by the rough waters of life. If some problems are like boulders dropped onto the starboard side of our little boats, causing us to list, we gain sixty pounds and plant ourselves portside to even things out. Sure, we've addressed the immediate problem, but at what cost?

Our princess had a boulder-size problem. During her newlywed years, her mirror told her one thing while her husband's lack of interest told her another. To address the imbalance, she changed her body until what she saw in the mirror lined up with the reality of her love-starved marriage. Bingo. Disparity solved, but at what price?

I know lots of women who have gained weight to balance out boat-rocking, boulder-size problems in their lives.

After being date-raped in college, Julia found herself feeling vulnerable around any man who was larger or stronger than she was. She doubled the size of her body, going from 125 pounds to nearly 250. Voilà. Problem solved, but at what cost?

Missy had fallen in love with a married man and, try as she might, was unable to walk away from the relationship. Her attraction to this man was tormenting and addicting at the same time. She remembers waking up one morning to the unbidden thought, "I know how to make this stop!" and the idea of gaining weight came to mind. Three months later she found herself forty pounds heavier — and her paramour moved on to shapelier pastures. She had solved her problem, but at what price?

I've known women who have put on weight to avoid affairs or to thumb their noses at controlling mothers. One woman I know needed time to heal after her divorce. She told me, "I keep trying to diet, but every time I lose ten pounds, I put it back on. I think it's because I'm not ready to date and my weight helps me tell the world, 'I'm not on the market. Leave me alone.' "

I said, "Gee whiz, can't you think of another way to take yourself off the market?"

The next day she went out and bought herself a fake wedding ring. She wore the ring for months and, lo and behold, suddenly eating healthier became a lot easier.

IS YOUR BODY AN ENEMY, OBJECT, OR FRIEND?

I wouldn't do something horrible to a friend just to solve a problem. I wouldn't, say, throw someone I loved in a rain-swollen gutter so I could keep my shoes dry as I stepped into the crosswalk.

I wouldn't ask a friend who wasn't hungry to eat a dozen donuts just to entertain me because I felt bored or restless.

I wouldn't even make a friend pay an exorbitant price to make my life a little easier. I wouldn't ask her, for example, to

176

write out a check for a thousand dollars so I wouldn't have to make an uncomfortable phone call or set a needed boundary with someone.

And I definitely wouldn't ask a friend to compromise her health so I could feel safe. I wouldn't ask her to gain fifty pounds and have acid reflux and high blood pressure just to save me the trouble of installing locks on my doors or taking a self-defense course or even going to counseling.

I love and respect my friends. I would never ask them to suffer just to spare me the work of finding a real solution to whatever dilemmas I may be facing. So why do I think it's okay to ask my body to pay that same price?

Maybe that's the problem. Maybe I don't think of my body as a friend. Perhaps I think of it as an enemy, or as someone who has betrayed me, or as something to be controlled. Anna Stookey, a bodymind psychotherapist who struggled with her own weight issues before finding a way through, describes in her blog similar realizations she came to about her body.[1]

I spent years dieting, running around, trying to do all the things I thought I was supposed to do to lose weight. I went to the gym three hours a day, tried all kinds of diets and fasts. I didn't sleep when I was tired or eat when I was hungry. Actually, I had no idea when I felt tired or hungry. I had completely stopped listening to — or loving — my body. I was trying to run my body like a well-organized to-do list.

Do you listen to your body, or have you gotten out of the habit of paying attention to the quiet signals it sends? I realized one day that it had been years — I mean actual years — since I'd experienced true hunger. I never felt light and empty anymore. The last time I'd heard my stomach growl, John Travolta was looking pretty hot in those white polyester disco pants he used to wear. I'd also resigned myself to suffering from heartburn every night and waking up every morning feeling sluggish and bloated. I wasn't seeing these "discomforts" as warning signs. I wasn't listening to my body as she shouted at me to stop shoveling in the food. My body was being overwhelmed by calories, manipulated by sugar, poisoned by preservatives, and buried beneath pounds of unwanted fat.

But despite our closeness — I mean, it's not like my body lives in another state — I couldn't hear a word she was screaming.

DEAR BODY . . .

Anna suggests, "When we think of our bodies as living, breathing things instead of objects to be controlled, our whole worldview changes." In her work as a bodymind psychotherapist, Anna often encourages clients to dialogue with their bodies as they move through health and weight issues. In her blog she tells the story of a client diagnosed with cancer who was about to begin treatment. "As his upcoming radiation loomed, we decided he should write a letter to his body about it. In the letter he would tell his body what the radiation was for, why he was doing it, and let his body know that it didn't have to fight against what was going to happen. He then pictured himself coming out of the treatment with no side effects — seeing himself in the waiting room following the procedure with an amazing amount of energy and appetite. He was actively communicating with his body to let it know what was about to happen as well as what he wanted the result to be." Anna reports that this client suffered virtually no side effects: he didn't lose weight, his hair, or his appetite. She wrote, "His doctors were stunned."

Even before hearing this story from Anna, I was starting to wonder if my body and I were overdue for a long heart-to-heart. Like Ricky Ricardo's zany wife, I had some 'splanin' to do. Had I, for years, been giving my body mixed signals and conflicting instructions? On the one hand, I'd asked my body to carry extra pounds to protect me from troubling emotions and further hurt. On the other hand, I'd hated her for being quick to accommodate my wishes. It was a wonder she was still speaking to me at all.

Maybe it was time to explain to my body what had been going on, as well as what changes I was ready to make. Feeling the need to clear the air — and maybe even release my body from the weird role of ballast to even out my emotions — I wrote these words in my journal:

> I want to tell my body that I don't hate her. That she's done well. I want to tell her "thank you" for protecting me all these years, but that it's not necessary anymore. I want her to know I'm going to be okay, that from now on I'm going to do whatever I need to do to find healthy solutions to my problems.

What might that look like? If I were going

to write a letter to my body, what might I say? What would you say to your body?

Here's what I'm telling my body: that I'm not going to use her as ballast to solve my problems anymore, that I'm sorry and that I'm beginning to understand how, without even meaning to, I gave her a terrible assignment many years ago, then hated her for faithfully following through with my request. She's not the enemy. She's been a loyal friend. I'm telling her "thank you" for her vigilance through the years, but that she has my permission to stop. I'm releasing her from the terrible assignment I put on her a very long time ago. I'm promising her that I'll figure things out. I'll set better boundaries. I'll learn to say no with my mouth and not my size. She can relax.

HEY, DO I KNOW YOU?

Whether you're rekindling a relationship or starting something new, it takes time to get to know each other. For several months I'd been making a real effort to treat my body well with healthy quantities of good food (instead of the sumo-wrestler quantities of junk food I'd been feeding her). One Sunday afternoon I found myself at an all-you-can-eat buffet with a pastor and his wife. Over the weekend I had spoken three times to the women in their church, and we were having lunch together before they took me to the airport. After months of healthy eating (and a busy weekend), I figured I deserved a reward. So as we walked into the restaurant, I told myself I could eat anything I wanted.

After giving myself permission to load my plate with whatever I felt like eating, I looked at my tray and was shocked at what I saw: A serving of baked fish. Broccoli. Long grain rice. A bowl of strawberries.

For the first time in my life I realized that — when I'm not confusing my body with massive amounts of carbs and calories — my body actually *likes* healthy food. Seriously, who knew?! Given permission to enjoy any mouth-watering item on that buffet — from sugar-dusted corn fritters to homemade mac and cheese to french silk pie — my body told me exactly what it wanted. And for the first time in years, I was listening.

If you're like a lot of women I know (myself included), you may start out eating healthy food and exercising because it's the right thing to do. But pretty soon, as all the junk-food noise in your body begins to subside, you may hear things you've never heard before. Like the still, small voice of reason, or the quiet hum of health and vitality, or even the grateful sigh of your very happy body. And the longer you turn your back on the clamoring din and pollution of junk-food living and embrace these quieter, simpler paths, the more aware you'll become of things your body has been trying to tell you all along.

A few months ago I was about to embark on a long hike with my daughters when it dawned on me that my muscles felt like they were made of lead. Having stopped for snacks at a small convenience store, I turned to Kacie and said, "I need a banana."

Since the store was fresh out of bananas, I spent the next ten minutes scanning labels on various bottles of sports drinks and juices. Eventually I bought a small carton of orange juice. The reason? Orange juice is full of potassium, which my heavy muscles were telling me I needed.

It felt like a small victory.

A couple of years ago I would never have heard my body's quiet request for potassium. How could I, when I wasn't paying attention to anything my body said?

Your body isn't your enemy. It's not ballast to be pumped up to counterbalance the weightier problems in life. It's not something to be controlled or hated or given weird subconscious assignments like getting all huge to protect you from stuff you really can learn how to handle.

If you've been at odds with your body, now's the time to make amends, even if you have to be the one to make the first move. Believe me, you're both going to feel a whole lot better.

GET A NEW BODITUDE

Questions for Personal Reflection or Group Discussion

- Do you give your body conflicting instructions? On the one hand, do you want your body to be healthy and shapely, but on the other hand do you adjust its size according to problems you need to solve in your life?

- What kinds of problems are most likely to send you scrambling for unhealthy solutions?

- Describe your relationship with your body. How do you treat each other? Can

---

you hear when your body is trying to tell you what she needs? And if you know what your body is asking for, do you try to give her what she needs or do you overrun the request with your own agenda?

• If you were to write a letter to your body, what would you say? In fact, I have a better idea. Use the space below to write that letter. Go ahead. Say what you need to say.

13

Even If You Don't Have the Body You'd Love, Love the One You Have

MAKING PEACE WITH YOUR LIFE TODAY

After working out for several months with Joe, I was feeling really good. I was breathing better and feeling stronger, more limber even. With progress like that, who wouldn't decide to try snowboarding?

Someone in her right mind, that's who.

I'm forty-nine. By now I've gotten used to being in control of my own limbs. I've also bought into the idea that hurtling myself unprotected through space may result in unpleasantness. Finally, I've watched enough hospital soap operas to know that intact bones are considered a good thing in most circumstances.

But my daughters had been begging for snowboard lessons for months, so when friends Gene and Belinda invited us to join them for a weekend at a ski resort in Angel Fire, New Mexico, how could I say no?

I couldn't. Which is fine. I didn't need to. What I *needed* to do was say no to snowboarding.

The first indication that I was in over my head should have been when our college-age instructor — who was on a first-name basis with all the other students, so you'd think he would have been calling me Karen — decided, instead, to call me Mom. If you're going to take up a new sport, consider it a red flag if your instructor takes one look at you and modifies his behavior based on his overwhelming awareness that he's young enough to be your offspring.

Over the next two hours, I was asked to take many of the natural instincts given to me at birth (instincts, by the way, that have been sharpened on the whetstones of wisdom and experience, such as the instinct to stay out of the ER) and throw them to the wind. Not that I saw much wind. Every time I got scared of going too fast on my snowboard, I wiped out. On purpose. Just took a dive and ploughed right into the snow, just to keep myself from picking up any unwanted speed and really hurting myself.

Later my instructor told me he'd never seen anyone wipe out from a complete standstill before.

I thought it was pretty cool, though, that I came home with a sports injury. That's when you know you've pushed the envelope and accomplished something beyond what you thought you'd ever do. So I was kind of proud of the fact that, for four days, my back and shoulders were so sore I could hardly turn over in bed. It gave me bragging rights. People would look at me and say, "You're walking funny," and I'd do the Barney Fife sniff and say, "Went snowboarding." Or someone would say, "Did you just groan reaching for that coffee pot?" and I'd say, "Oh that? Snowboarding." They'd say "Did you want fries with that order?" and I'd say nonchalantly, "Yep. Snowboarding."

Although, to be honest, I'm not sure I actually got hurt snowboarding. I might have done it getting off the chairlift. There was this small incident where I tried to hop off the chair but forgot to let go. Next thing I knew, the chair had knocked me flat and was dragging me through the snow. People were really helpful, though. A bunch of them stood around and shouted, "Let go of the chair! LET GO OF THE CHAIR!"

Maybe I spoke too quickly about never snowboarding again. At least it created some wonderful memories for me and my daughters. I think the problem was that I got overzealous and signed up for the wrong class. Next time I'll start with something better suited to my skill level.

Can anyone point me to the line for chair-lift lessons?

BETTER NOW THAN NEVER

Is it ever really too late to try something new? Or too late to get in shape?

One day I called my mom and said, "Break out the spandex because I'm bringing Joe to your house tomorrow morning for your first workout!" This grandmother of eight not only agreed, she was ecstatic! My mom will be the first to tell you that she's never been particularly athletic, although she does walk in her neighborhood on nice days, and last year she joined a gym and worked out for several weeks before spraining her wrist on one of the machines.

After our first workout, she noticed a difference. "Wow! I feel energized!" she bubbled. "I feel stronger! My joints feel looser!"

As Joe says, "See? It's never too late to start exercising."

Indeed, the myth that, at some point in our lives, we get too old to enjoy the benefits of activity is long dead. One study, published in the *British Journal of Sports Medicine,* concludes that staying aerobically fit through middle age and beyond can delay biological aging by up to twelve years.[1] Another study, by Drs. Tarnopolsky and Melov at the Buck Institute for Age Research, documented that six months of resistance training can reverse some of the changes in muscle tone and metabolism caused by aging.[2] Still other studies prove that older adults who exercise get a boost in brainpower, improving memory and focus and helping them process information faster. Additional benefits of exercise for adults of every age, according to Joe, include reduced risks of serious disease, faster recovery after injury or illness, better sleep, and reduced risks of falls.

Joe adds that if you want to stay healthy and independent at any age, the National Institutes of Health recommends four kinds of exercise:

- strength training, which builds muscles, increases your metabolism rate, and helps keep your weight and blood sugar in check
- stretching exercises, which encourage greater freedom of movement
- endurance exercises such as walking, jogging, biking, or swimming, which help control weight, prevent heart

disease, and increase blood circulation
- balance exercises, which build leg muscles and help prevent falls

As Joe explained to Mom and me, "Balance exercises don't get the respect they deserve. Weight training and cardio are great because they work large muscle groups, but they miss the small stabilizing muscles that improve balance and stability. These small muscles are the ones that help us avoid falls and injuries, which is important through our entire lives but especially as we age."

My mom has so much confidence in the benefits of exercise that she's been trying to get my dad to lift weights with us. So far he's managed to avoid the workouts. He says he's strong enough already, and the man may have a point. He's seventy-five and can still lift printing presses and large farm animals without breaking a sweat. Although if he's this strong at his age without working out, think what he could do if he committed to regular cardio and weight training.

I'll bet he could do anything! Even snowboard.

I HAD TO FALL IN LOVE WITH ME

It was June 3, 1959, and five-year-old Mary McManus had just gotten vaccinated the previous day to protect her against polio. She told me, "I was in gym class and dancing around the room with the other kindergarteners when I just dropped."

I said, "Dropped? From pain? From fatigue?"

"No. I was paralyzed."

Surgery followed, as did rehabilitative therapy. Mary remembers, "I was five and my physical therapist read Dr. Seuss to me before every painful session, and we quoted lines from the book to each other as she worked on me, trying to retrain my muscles."

Mary's paralysis was on the left side of her body. She says she was lucky — many people who contracted polio in the 1950s died; others ended up in iron lungs. Eventually she regained a portion of her mobility, married, and enjoyed a career in social work. But she still hated the skin she was in. She says, "I survived polio, but I hated my body. I felt it had betrayed me with the polio virus. I saw my body as something to be tolerated as I literally and metaphorically limped through life. As wonderful as my doctor and rehab therapists were back in the fifties, I never learned that my body is sacred because it holds *me*."

When Mary was fifty-two, she began suffering with new muscle weakness, pain, and fatigue and was eventually diagnosed with post-polio syndrome (PPS). PPS can go undetected for years, showing up several decades after someone first contracted the disease. Finding herself back in a leg brace and using a cane and sometimes a wheelchair, Mary was beyond discouraged. And when doctors and therapists told her she'd have to quit the job she loved in order to manage her new symptoms, she felt her world had come to an end.

Mary had no idea what to do next or what her purpose was supposed to be. After pouring herself into her work for twenty-five years, she was cut loose. Now she had even more reasons to loathe her body, which seemed more broken than ever before.

That's when she turned to God.

"I'd always had a faith and a relationship with God," Mary explains, "but, like any relationship, sometimes it's stronger than at other times, and sometimes you get distracted. Well, I'd been busy for years with my kids and career, and I'd forgotten how important it is to stay connected to God. Getting post-polio syndrome reminded me how much I needed that relationship."

One afternoon, after crying out to God about her fears and concerns, Mary got up, limped to her laptop, and began to write. Verses poured out of her like water, and she titled her poem "Running the Race." More poetry began to follow. But these poems weren't humorous, like the Seuss verses that had soothed her when she was five years old. And they weren't like the fun verses Mary had written for her kids when they were in school, celebrating birthdays or special events in their lives.

Mary says, "Suddenly, everything I was writing was about my relationship with my body."

She remembers, "During that time, I was often in a wheelchair and was just happy when I could get out of the chair and walk from point A to point B. But suddenly I began to write about running a race, about seeing my body running in a 10K. Through poetry, I began to experience the wonder and freedom of my body. It was a paradox because my body was immobilized, yet my spirit was feeling so happy and free. It created this whole new view of my body. For the first time, I was able to say to my body, like Mr. Rogers, 'I love you just the way you are.'

"I bought a bright blue cane. I began saying to myself, *You know what? These polio shoes are beautiful. Who cares if I can't wear high heels?* I began to see myself as whole and healthy. It didn't matter what the outcome was — whether I would ever get around without a leg brace or cane or wheelchair — I still needed to feel whole and healthy in my own skin."

As she began to love and accept her body for the first time, Mary's body began to respond in new ways to therapy and then to a fitness program designed for her by a close friend and personal trainer, Janine Hightower.[3] Mary was able to abandon the leg brace and, over the following year, continued gaining strength. Miraculously, she went on to train for — and finish! — the Boston Marathon as a mobility-impaired runner, completing 26.2 miles alongside her husband and daughter and raising $10,535 for polio research.

Mary remembers what it was like to approach the finish line. The professional athletes and front runners were long gone, but Boylston Street was still lined with people, cheering and cheering. Mary saw her son and her personal trainer and hundreds of other faces.

Seven hours and forty-two minutes after

she began, Mary crossed the line. She could barely stand. Her legs were spent. When a volunteer came to untie the timing chip from Mary's shoe, she could barely keep her balance. The man told her, "Lean on me," as he knelt to remove the chip. When he stood up, there were tears in his eyes and he hugged her.

Today Mary says, "Three years ago I thought I'd lost my purpose. Since then, I've published one book of poetry and am completing my second book. I blog about celebrating the blessing of — finally! — being able to love every inch of this body that has gone through so much and still needs extra-tender care to manage all my symptoms. My story has been on the news and in a documentary, and I've gotten to speak to many different groups. My passion and purpose is to let people who are dealing not only with PPS but with other neurological diseases know that . . . there is always hope and possibility. And when you love yourself, that's when the magic and miracles happen."[4]

LIFE DOESN'T BEGIN WHEN I'M THIN

Here's another question: While it's never too late to learn how to love ourselves, our bodies, and our lives . . . can it ever be *too soon?* I can't tell you how often I've heard women say, "As soon as I lose some weight I'm going to _____." You can fill in the blank. Everything from attend a class reunion, make hotter love to their husbands, get their belly buttons pierced, take the kids to the pool, go on vacation, join a gym, and even get a new do. (And I'm *really* not going to tell you how often the woman saying this sort of thing has been me.)

It's way too easy to keep putting life on hold, waiting for something to happen before we start loving our bodies, loving ourselves, and loving our lives.

Have you ever put your life on hold because you are uncomfortable with your body? Danielle says she fell into that category until she started doing two things that moved her into what she calls the "now I love and accept my body" category. Here are the two things she did:

She started attending yoga classes regularly.

She started wearing comfortable, beautiful clothing regardless of the number on her scale.

None of this "I don't *care* if nothing fits, I *refuse* to buy anything new until I lose weight!" for this girl! I love Danielle's wardrobe 'tude, especially since apparently she travels up and down the scale about as often as I do, making sure she's got a week's worth of work clothes in every size from 8 to 20. She told me, "No matter what I weigh, wearing the right-size clothes is part of how I stopped warring with my shape and figure. My self-confidence increases when I refuse to try to hide my body inside clothes that are baggy and shapeless. And my comfort and happiness increase when I refuse to try to squeeze myself into things that leave me in pain, pinched, out of breath, or with big red marks gouged into my skin at the end of the day."

And I love her insights regarding the yoga class she attends. She wrote to me, "Going to class and seeing people of all shapes and sizes doing the poses and struggling just like I do was a huge part of loving and accepting my body. It also helped me feel like I was truly *in* my body. I used to feel like 'I' was only in my mind and separate from my body. But suddenly I began to realize my body wasn't a separate thing that was doing things to me (and vice versa). I began to feel integrated and more whole."

"THIS IS THE MOMENT . . . MY PERFECTION"

How do we begin to make peace with our lives today? Perhaps it begins when we stop focusing on what we've never had, what we no longer possess, or even what we have yet to attain — and start living as fully as we can with whatever we have *right now*.

In chapter 4, I quoted a woman named Jeacline who wrote to me: "I've been on diets since I was seven. I'm not sure how it started, but I always saw myself as fat! Now it seems ridiculous to me." Those words were just a snippet of her letter. Now I'd like to let her share the rest of her story:[5]

Hello Karen,

I'm 43, 5'2", 135 lbs and got colon cancer about a year and a half ago. I'm still here, fighting it. And I'm so grateful for my body!

I've been on diets since I was seven. I'm not sure how it started, but I always saw myself as fat! Now it seems ridiculous to me. Seriously! How can 135 lbs be fat?

I don't know why I thought I was fat. Of course, 135 isn't lean exactly. I mean, I have a bit of padding here and there. But I now look at myself in the mirror, with my long sexy swaying scar and all, and I get an involuntary smile on my face and whisper a thank you to whoever, not even sure, since I don't believe in God anymore. Old habit, I guess . . .

I think back a few years ago and how critical I was of myself. Every inch, every freckle, every little cushion and skin spot, was irritating to me. I wanted perfection and didn't even know that I had it already! I had a perfect little body, healthy and strong and completely intact. And I was ungrateful still.

I'm grateful now and happy to show it off. Tastefully of course. But I feel no shame or embarrassment or shyness when I get naked in front of my man anymore. I don't have thoughts of *I can't let him see me in that position because I will look fat* anymore. I wear my clothes proudly now. Before, I would always wear long sleeves because I thought my arms were fat. I wore a sleeveless summer dress last weekend, and my arms were just lovely and so happy to be out and be seen! My belly is still a bit swollen from my last surgery a couple of weeks ago, but that's okay; my dress was a bit loose and I looked so lovely in it.

My hair isn't always styled nowadays;

some days are just harder to get through. And I'm not embarrassed to let people see me this way. I can run errands and even meet with clients "au naturel," so to speak, and I'm ok with that because it's me. I'm beautiful just as I am and don't have to enhance myself to allow others to see me. The natural me is good enough for them too.

I'm grateful because I know I look and feel better than I ever will in the future, however long my future turns out to be.

This is the moment. This is my perfection. We're always changing and we're always getting older. We forget that in five or ten or fifteen years, we won't look or feel as good as now. Now is the best time of our lives. Now is the youngest we'll ever be, the healthiest we'll ever be, the best looking we'll ever be.

I've shared my thoughts with many of my dear friends, male and female, young and old, and I am seeing a difference in how they think and feel about their bodies, their looks. . . .

I don't know why I got cancer; I've lived a healthier lifestyle than *any* of the people I know. They are all a bit shocked and scared by the fact that cancer can strike someone like me. But this is one of the benefits of cancer for me: to love myself more just as I am, and maybe this can be something I can turn into a gift to others, to share my regrets about not having loved myself more in the past, when I was even more beautiful and healthy and "perfect." . . . I continue to talk about it, to keep reminding everyone not to waste time in self-criticism but to love themselves just as they are now, while, of course, always striving to be healthier in mind, spirit, *and* body.

I suspect this isn't what you would call "dieting success," but in many ways this is the *most* effective "diet" I've ever been on. It's just a different kind of diet. It's a diet of the mind, getting rid of all the excess negative self-talk, dissatisfaction, and ungratefulness, and choosing instead to be happy and grateful for what we've got, appreciating what we have so much that we want to do things to keep it healthy and strong, like eating healthier and moving more and sleeping enough and not working too much and showing pride in it and being kind to it. . . .

I hope that I've given you food for thought yourself. If you are like the average woman, you may have things you are unsatisfied in and about yourself. Stop

202

it. You are the best you're ever going to be. Be grateful and appreciate what you've got. I hope you've never been stricken with a terminal illness, and I hope that you can learn something from the wisdom that comes to only those who have. Be so very grateful and love yourself just as you are.

Blessings to you,
Jeacline

Dear Jeacline,

I was going to end my chapter here, with your words. I figured you said it best, and there would be nothing more to add.

And, in a way, there's not.

Except for this.

Thank you.

It wasn't until just now, just this minute, reading your letter for the third or fourth time — but this time reading it slowly, for the last time before sending this particular chapter off to my editor — that I noticed something I hadn't noticed before.

I saw how personal you made your last paragraph. Maybe it escaped me until now because earlier in your letter you talked about sharing your story with lots of people, anyone who will listen, really. So for some reason, every time I read your closing words, I kept seeing them the same way, as a message for the masses.

And they are, of course. But I saw just now that you didn't actually write those words to the masses. You wrote them to me. And as that sunk in, really sunk in, my eyes filled with tears because . . . well . . . I needed that.

Trust me, I write books like this not because I know all the answers, but because I know all the questions. And I know the questions because I wrestle with them, every day, in the private world of my own doubts and insecurities. And I've been wrestling really hard lately, and lately I've been tasting my own sweat and tears on the mat more often than I'd like to admit.

But I'm going to listen to you. I am going to stop it. I'm going to learn from your wisdom and make a choice to be grateful and appreciate who I am and what I have today. I'm even going to copy the words from that paragraph, the words you wrote to me, and put them on my mirror where I can see them every day.

And, Jeacline, I don't know what happened between you and God, but I do know that sometimes we believe, then stuff happens, then we stop believing. I've even been there myself. Sometimes — and I know this too — something begins to stir, and we find it in our hearts to believe again.

If you find this happening to you, would you do something for me? Would you allow yourself to see where it leads you? Sometimes faith crashes and burns and, as with the phoenix, something beautiful that once took flight gets reduced to nothing but memories and ash. But sometimes a wind kicks up, and the ashes stir and then begin to dance. And if we're quiet and still, and willing to be surprised, we just might find ourselves in awe at what happens next.

Gratefully yours,

Karen

GET A NEW BODITUDE

Questions for Personal Reflection or Group Discussion

• What is keeping you from getting started on changing your life? What are *you* waiting for?

• Like Mary, do you feel there are ways in which your body has betrayed you? Is there something you can do that will help you stop resenting your body for what it can't do, and begin appreciating it for what it *can* do?

• If you had the body of your dreams, how would you live your life differently than you do now? What might happen if you made a decision to go ahead and start living parts of that life now?

- If you went on a "diet of the mind," as Jeacline suggests, what might that look like? Jeacline got rid of negative self-talk, dissatisfaction, and ungratefulness. What would you choose to lose?

14

IF THEY'RE NOT SEXY, WHY ARE THEY CALLED LOVE HANDLES?

MAKING PEACE WITH SEX

You know you're not comfortable with your body when your husband, away on a business trip, calls you one night and says in his most husky, turned-on voice, "What are you wearing?" and you say "Sweat pants and an overcoat."

For many women, the thought of getting naked for anything other than showering (by themselves) is enough to make them want to step in front of a bus. How we look naked — not to mention how we *think* we look and especially how we think our *husbands* think we look — is a big deal. I don't know too many women who have not struggled with this issue.

And yet, sex doesn't have to make us feel bad about our bodies, and our bodies don't need to make us feel insecure about making love. That is, if we can just grasp a couple of important concepts. This is because the way we feel about sex and the way sex makes us feel about ourselves may be influenced less by the shape of our bodies than by the health of our body attitudes. We need to develop better boditudes.

What kind of boditudes do you embrace? What new ones should you consider? Here are several concepts that have made a real difference in my life.

WANTED: GREAT BODY IMAGE (GREAT BODY OPTIONAL)

A number of years ago I was part of a small group of women that met weekly. The group members were interested in adding sparkle to their marriages, and while nary a one of us would have turned down a diamond of any kind, that's not exactly the kind of sparkle we were aiming for.

One evening a woman mentioned a romantic getaway during which she had enjoyed performing a strip tease for her husband. Another woman, with a mixture of disbelief and admiration in her voice, asked, "Weren't you self-conscious? How could you do that? I could never do that."

What struck me was that the woman who'd been happy to strut her stuff was fifty pounds overweight, while the woman who would rather undergo a root canal had the figure of a swimsuit model. Our insecurities about our bodies can be rogue emotions, functioning independent of minor details like . . . um . . . reality. Meaning we can look like Eva Mendes and still feel like Marge Simpson.

That's the bad news.

The good news is that the reverse is also true. We can look like Marge and still feel as sexy and confident as Eva. A healthy body image begins in the head, not on the scale.

I'm struggling with this right now. Sometimes the numbers on my scale resemble the stock market, up one day, down the next. (If I could just get my numbers to stick to resembling the stock market during a recession, I'd be a lot happier.) My point is, when I give in to defeatist thinking, I'm a lot more likely to give up, letting my emotional eating have its cruel way with me. But when I fight that urge — when I remind myself that feeling good about my body is a function of my head, not my waistline — it's easier to see my added pounds as a temporary condition rather than as a defining flaw.

SEXY IS IN THE EYE
OF THE BEHOLDER

Your husband thinks you're sexier than you think he does. According to an article titled "10 Mistakes Women Make When Having Sex," a common misconception that many women buy into is *thinking her man feels the way about her body that she does.* The author, Rod Phillips (note: *Rod,* as in "this is a man writing this and not a woman simply engaging in wishful thinking"), had this to say on the subject:

> Men don't attach the judgments to women's bodies that women do. So, for example, even if he thinks your butt really is a bit on the large side, it won't matter to him the way it matters to you. In fact, he probably quite likes it. And he certainly won't be put off making love, or want the lights off, because of it. While you waste time and emotional energy wondering if you're completely undesirable because of some aspect of your body, he'll never give it a second thought. It's women who judge their bodies, I think for the sake of comparison with other women, not men.[1]

We may think we need perfect bodies to

have great sex, but maybe it works like this: while our husbands might love our bodies to be perfect, they'd also like to have superhero powers and drive Lamborghinis, but they know they're not going to get those things either.

If Rod is to be believed, smart men come to terms with these little disappointments, going on to enjoy perfectly happy mortal lives driving Chevrolets and making sweet love to sexy, imperfect women.

SEXY IS ABOUT PASSION, NOT PERFECTION

As a single woman, I've gotten to know a number of single men, some as dates and some as friends. More often than not, if a guy is sharing with me the Cliffs Notes version of the stuff that accompanied the demise of his marriage, he says something like this: "She never wanted to have sex because . . . ," or, "She would never undress in front of me because . . . ," and the next phrase is usually a variation of "she thought she was too fat" or "she thought her hips were too big."

I usually ask, "Was she?" or, "Were they?" Often the answer is, "No way! I loved her body!" Or, "It didn't bother me as much as it bothered her" or, "What I *really* wanted was for her to be excited about our sex life, for her to want to be with me as much as I wanted to be with her."

Granted, I have yet to interview the ex-wives. But the stories I get from ex-husbands ring true. I say this because I also talk to women, married and divorced, who tell me the same story from the other side of the coin. My friend Barb expressed it well: "Robert is as amorous as ever, but I can't go there. If I'm honest with myself, the thirty pounds I gained aren't responsible for derailing our love life. My *inhibitions* over those thirty pounds, however, have left my guy feeling frustrated and abandoned."

My friend Jackie told me this next story, which I love. Like many of us, Jackie would like to lose some pounds. The extra weight not only robs her of energy, but it gets in the way of feeling sexy. Oh, her husband doesn't complain, but Jackie spends a good part of their lovemaking feeling more embarrassed than aroused.

One day while helping her twelve-year-old daughter with a homework assignment, Jackie gained a new perspective that culminated in a whole new lease on love. She explains:

Melissa was doing a research paper on

the seventeenth-century painter Paul Rubens. He's famous for painting naked, buxom, glowing women of the Renaissance. (Buxom, in fact, might be putting it mildly.) Anyway, as Melissa and I were going through a library book filled with photos of his paintings, it struck me that the women he painted — considered beautiful in his day and in ours as well — were fat. They had thunder thighs and thick waists and rolling bosoms, and they were sensuous and confident and beautiful. The more I looked at his work, the more I began to think about myself. Maybe I could be sensuous and confident and beautiful too.

That night Jackie had the chance to put her hypothesis to the test. She says she was less inhibited and more adventurous than she'd been in years. Afterward her husband summed up the experience with a simple "Wow!"

Later, curled in the crook of his arm, Jackie told her husband about the revelation that had changed her perspective and helped to begin to accept her body with all of its voluptuous, comfortable curves. When she finished her story, her husband kissed her tenderly on top of her head and said,

"Maybe you should help Melissa with her homework more often."

SEXY WOMEN DON'T COMPARE THEMSELVES TO FICTIONAL CHARACTERS

Apparently, while a guy may be able to accept the fact that he is *not* married to Angelina Jolie, what he can't accept is being married to a woman who refuses to enthusiastically make love to him because her body doesn't look like Angie's or Demi's or Cameron's.

Which reminds me. There's a distinct possibility that even Angie, Demi, and Cameron don't look like Angie, Demi, and Cameron. This is because Hollywood's roster of image magicians contains not only airbrush artists but also "body part models." These are men and women who make a living modeling parts of their bodies as doubles for actors and actresses. Let's say your favorite actress appears in a movie that includes a scene requiring a closeup on her hands. It's entirely possible that the flawless digits you see on your TV screen are not those of the celebrated actress but the pampered palms of a hand model. And it's not just hands. Thighs, breasts, and derrières are up for grabs as well. (Figuratively speaking, of course.)

When I learned about this aspect of Hollywood trickery, it made me mad. For years I have been comparing myself unfavorably to the flickering images of flawless womanhood on the silver screen, only to find out that these icons of perfection don't exist. Even all the moneybags and power moguls of Hollywood can't locate in one woman all of the "best" physical amenities. So they create a celluloid composite of the choicest features and present them to society as the ideal woman.

The hard reality is that a hot new starlet might very well have wrinkled hands, while the fill-in hand model with flawless fingers is equipped with Hindenburg hips. You and I only get to view (and compare ourselves to) the finished product: the perfect composite woman. Frankenstein would be proud.

So don't be so hard on yourself. You are not a second-class woman because your hands sweat or you have morning breath or you've gained a few pounds.

SEXY WOMEN ENJOY FULL LIVES

I once met a woman who bragged she still had pert, firm breasts after nursing four babies. Four babies? Perky breasts? It's not that I don't believe her but . . . if she told me the sun was shining in July, I'd be tempted to want a second opinion. Some things — including pregnancy, childbirth, nursing, and the passing of years — take a toll on a woman's body. We end up with stretch marks, widened hips, and tired breasts. Caring for a young family can mean dark circles from sleepless nights, dishpan hands, and a permanent squint from driving into the sun as you carpool fourteen hours each week. Raising teens? Say hello to worry wrinkles, premature gray, and arthritic fingers from spending eight years gripping your wallet tightly in a futile, protective gesture.

A few years back I took a long look at my hands and was surprised to see that the smooth, taut skin of my youth had been changed. So maybe my skin is not as supple as it once was, but I also have a family and a career and a couple of dogs. I have things to do and people to love. I'm guessing I've passed the halfway mark of my allotted years on this earth, and I've got the scars and the laugh lines to prove it.

There's a saying "age before beauty." But what's wrong with having both? At every age we are sexy and beautiful as we learn to appreciate, respect, and cherish the sacrifices our bodies make as we pursue all the wonderful things our lives have to offer.

SEXY IS AS SEXY DOES

One day this subject came up with a counselor I was seeing during my marriage. For some reason I happened to be by myself on the day of this particular session. As the counselor and I talked, I told him that I sometimes felt my body wasn't perfect enough for me to feel as confident during sex as I wanted to. What he said in response struck home with me. He said: "Sex isn't *static* art. It's not like a photo or sculpture that's meant to be studied and admired. Sex is *performance* art, and I'm not talking about performance in terms of faking something. Performance art, like a fabulous dance, is dynamic. It is rhythm and life and movement. And that's what makes it beautiful."

His perspective made *so* much sense to me!

According to sex educator and relationship expert Dr. Yvonne Fulbright, "A big complaint you'll hear from men and women alike is that their lover didn't do much of anything during sex. Men have grumbled that she doesn't move during lovemaking. Most people like an active lover — one responsive to the action, which shows that they're into the moment."[2]

Enjoyment, like laughter or movement, is contagious. When two people are immersed in intimate enjoyment of each other, evaluating the thickness of a thigh or the wattle on an arm isn't nearly as important as it seems when you're by yourself evaluating your imperfections.

SEXY IS A TEAM SPORT

It's easy to fall into the trap of thinking sex is about how we look, but it's not. It's about reaching beyond ourselves — past facades, past skin even — and creating a bridge from "one" to "two becoming one." Sex isn't about striking the right pose, but about creating a meaningful connection. We can lose sight of this when we shift our focus to what we see in the mirror.

Sex is synergy. And as we see it that way — as something to create rather than something we have to measure up to — we may very well find ourselves enjoying new vistas in our relationships with our husbands and in our relationships with our own bodies as well.

GET A NEW BODITUDE

Questions for Personal Reflection or Group Discussion

• Does the prospect of making love cause you to feel bad about your body? Does the way you feel about your body make you feel insecure about making love? Why or why not?

• Some men say that a woman who is comfortable in her own skin is about as sexy as it gets. What are your thoughts?

• What is holding you back from loving your love life and your body? Dynamics in your relationship with your husband? Past hurts? Unrealistic expectations?

• What steps can you take to break free from issues that prevent you from making peace with this part of your life?

15

WILL WORK FOR CHOCOLATE

MAKING PEACE WITH YOUR CRAVINGS

My doctor said something weird the other day. He told me to eat more real food. I thought it was strange because, you know, it's not like I'm five years old and eating imaginary cookies. I told him I *do* eat real food and I can prove it. I grabbed the tire around my waist and said, "You don't get *this* from make-believe tea parties!"

But he might be onto something. Have you ever thought about the things you and I crave? If you're like me, the stuff that calls your name usually falls into the *faux* food category, in the company of things that don't exist in nature, such as chicken fingers and curly fries. I'm thinking if 90 percent of what I eat comes from a factory and not from a field or a farm, it's probably not a good thing.

We're making a lot of headway, you and me. We've accepted the idea that yo-yo diets aren't the answer. We're making small changes and learning new approaches to food and even keeping food journals. We're getting more exercise and being more intentional regarding the feelings and beliefs we embrace about ourselves. We're practicing better habits, making friends with our emotions, and broadening our definition of beauty. We're even going to stop being so hard on ourselves and start having more fun during sex!

But some days we still turn into vacuum cleaners with teeth. What's up with that?

Maybe it wouldn't be such a problem if we craved healthy things like celery and tofu. Or if our cravings didn't make us chubby or cause us to feel out of control and pathetic. This isn't a book about reducing calories, but it *is* a book about changing our bodies, loving ourselves, and transforming our lives. And that includes learning how to manage the cravings that leave us feeling fat, pathetic, and powerless.

What's Fat Got to Do with It?

One Saturday I felt cranky, tired, and hungry. After spending half the day eating salads and struggling to stay awake, I gave up and headed to my room for a nap, grabbing a handful of M&M's on the way.

I woke up a few hours later feeling even hungrier. I was scurrying back to the kitchen for more M&M's when I remembered Joe's saying something about fat having the ability to satiate hunger, so I veered toward the fridge to grab the jar of natural peanut butter. Doling out two tablespoons of the golden goo, I ate it spread over a half-dozen stalks of celery. And for the first time all day, I began to feel a little better.

Since then I've learned that a moderate serving of fat slows down digestion, meaning our stomachs get empty more slowly, meaning we feel full longer than if we'd eaten only carbs or protein.

Could something I'm *not* eating be fueling my cravings?

A lot of times, when we're dieting, we go to the market and fill our carts with fat-free versions of all our favorite foods. Fat-free ice cream, hot dogs, cookies, milk, yogurt, cheese. I've even bought fat-free half-n-half, which seems like the ultimate oxymoron. The point is, we think we're doing ourselves a favor, but are we really? If a moderate serving of fat helps satiate hunger, no wonder fat-free knockoffs have a hard time leaving us satisfied! Plus, when manufacturers pull the fat out of products, they usually have to replace it with something else in order to maintain texture or flavor. That's why fat-free foods can be higher in things like calories, sodium, or carbs.

I wonder if a tiny bit of real sugar doesn't help as well. This is because, at least for me, twenty cups of tea sweetened with artificial sweetener won't quell my cravings as well as a single cup of tea sweetened with a spoonful of honey.

It's dawning on me that real foods are all right — even helpful — if consumed in moderation. And, according to Joe, the key word here is *moderation.* Meaning downing a spoonful of peanut butter is a good thing, while downing a half carton of ice cream is not.

Who knew?

TAKE A CHILL PILL

Diana Walker calls herself a cravings coach, and, indeed, her Web site offers a smorgasbord of information and practical tips for quelling the cravings that drive us nuts. She says that whether we're stressed or relaxed while we're eating may make the difference when it comes to food cravings and even weight loss.[1]

She writes, "One of the major reasons you experience cravings is because your body isn't properly using the nutrients that it is receiving," adding that eating in front of the television, eating while we're stressed, or even eating quickly can hinder our bodies from absorbing the things they need, leading to more hunger and cravings later.

How do we lower our stress level or calm our emotions during mealtimes? Here are some tips from Diana:

- Start by having real "sit-down" meals. When you take the time to relax while you are eating, you'll be able to enjoy your food and digest it as well.
- When you eat a meal or a snack, slow down so you can get maximum enjoyment from eating. Don't rush!
- Pay attention to your emotions. If you eat on the run or when you're feeling sad, angry, or stressed, you'll end up having food cravings shortly afterward. If you're in the middle of a bunch of crazy emotions — feeling overwhelmed, sad, mad, or even just bored and restless — first do something that

225

will help you relax *before* you have your next meal. Diana suggests trying meditation and other relaxation techniques.

She writes, "If you've never meditated before, it may seem intimidating. Really it's nothing more than just sitting in a quiet spot and focusing your attention on something fixed. Some people try to think of one word like 'peace,' and others try to clear their mind entirely. It's up to you to find what's most pleasing and relaxing for you. The point is to find a method that helps you get your mind off of food and on to what is really important, your relaxation."[2]

You and I are binge savvy enough to know that crazy emotions make us eat crazy (that's why it's called "emotional eating"). We already know that when we're feeling stressed, upset, or bored and reaching for food, there's a good chance we're going to eat too much of a lot of very wrong things.

But even for an experienced binge master like myself, Diana's words are revealing. In the past, I've thought that — in order to defuse emotional eating — I had to get to the root of the emotions driving my frantic foray through the pantry. If I was anxious about finances, for example, I figured I needed to not only work through my anxiety, but also reorganize my budget, get a second job, and invite all my creditors to my home for a group hug before I'd be truly free to pass up the four boxes of Girl Scout cookies.

In other words, I've been under the impression that to stop emotional eating, I needed to solve the problem that was fueling the emotion that was driving my eating. Which is trying to pack a lot into the two minutes it takes me to grab a plate, checkered bib, and utensils and plant myself at the kitchen table for a serious chow-down. Which is why Diana's words are freeing. Maybe I don't have to solve the problem that's driving my emotions before I can step away from the food. Maybe all I need to do right now is *relax.*

In chapter 9, I mentioned relaxation as one of the techniques that is highly touted in addiction-recovery groups for managing cravings. After reading Diana's insights, it's easy to see why. She suggests meditation as a way to relax, which makes me think of something I frequently do before meals, which is pause in prayer. In those brief moments, I thank God for taking care of my daughters and me and for providing the food we're about to eat.

Are you and I missing an opportunity here? What if we did more than just pause for thirty seconds to thank God for our food? What if we took five minutes, even ten, and just sat quietly in his presence? What if we were completely silent? What if we just sat with grateful hearts and listened? What might he whisper to us, what words of encouragement or comfort or direction might we hear? What if we imagined taking all the stresses and problems of our day and laying them in a tidy bundle at God's feet? What if we imagined emptying our hearts of everything except contentment and gratitude and an awareness of his presence?

I don't know about you, but that would feel a lot different to me than the thirty-second acknowledgement I typically toss his way before picking up my fork. If I could relax in God's presence and fix my attention on him and his care for me, I'd go into my meal feeling a lot different. I'm guessing I'd have a greater awareness of feeling centered and even loved. I'd probably feel less needy too. And I'd definitely feel less alone.

Let's give it a try.

A GRAB BAG OF CRAVING SOLUTIONS

What else can stop a craving dead in its tracks? Different things work for different people, which is why I asked several dozen women about the strategies they use when they need to stop shoveling things into their mouths. Here's what they came up with, along with my further comments:

- Brush your teeth. Put on your teeth-whitening strips if you have to! It'll keep you from putting food in there.
- Drink a big glass of water. As Joe says, sometimes that "I need something, I just don't know what it is" feeling isn't signaling true hunger, but *thirst.* To alleviate thirst-driven hunger, stay hydrated. You'll find yourself spending less time standing in front of the open fridge door hunting for something to satisfy that unidentifiable urge.
- Eat carbs that are high in fiber. When your body needs fuel, the first thing it burns is the carbohydrates you consumed most recently. And yet, not all carbs are created equal. Some carbs turn to sugar slowly in your body, making you feel satisfied longer and providing a steady level of energy. Other carbs turn to sugar quickly, giving you

a burst of energy and then dropping you sharply back into hunger. To feel full longer and enjoy a steadier level of energy, Joe recommends choosing slow-burning carbs such as brown rice, whole-grain breads, and colorful, fiber-rich fruits and veggies such as red and yellow peppers, spinach, and yams. Avoid processed carbs such as white bread, white rice, potatoes, bagels, and white tortillas. In other words, don't eat white.

- Get six or more hours of sleep each night. When you sleep less than six hours a night, your sleep-deprived body produces less leptin, a blood protein that suppresses appetite and helps your brain know when you've had enough food. To make matters worse, sleep-starved bodies produce additional grehlin which stimulates your appetite, tempting you to ramp up the calories the following day. By sleeping a minimum of six hours every night, you can avoid setting up a chain of responses in your body that will sabotage you the following day.
- Get out of the house and kitchen. Go for a walk or take a drive.
- Ask yourself how long it has been since

you've eaten. Like Michelle in chapter 6, maybe your cravings are a sign of true hunger. If so, eat a healthy meal.

- Take your vitamins. There may be nutrients you are missing and, if so, a supplement may help.
- Have healthy snacks prepared and ready to go. Keep salsa on hand, which is a great, low-calorie snack, but nix the chips and try carrot sticks instead. (One woman said that enjoying salsa right from a spoon sometimes helps quench her nibbles!) Keep celery, bell peppers, marinated portabella mushrooms, grapes, and oranges on hand and ready to eat.
- Find something else to do with your hands. Knit, garden, scrapbook, or wash dishes. It's hard to shovel stuff in your mouth when your hands are busy.

I must admit that keeping your hands occupied is not a foolproof strategy against snacking. I recently posted a question on Facebook: "If you're writing on the computer and eating popcorn at the same time, how can you keep the butter off your keyboard?"

Jene suggested drinking my popcorn from a cup, Bronwyn told me to type with my elbows, and Bonnie advised wiping my hands on my jeans. Diane thought I should stop typing and just go for the popcorn.

Geoffrey was the most creative, offering detailed instructions and even diagrams for a complex pulley system that would allow me to tip popcorn from a storage container over my head, funneling it into my mouth while wearing a postsurgery doggie cone around my neck. That way, the popcorn wouldn't fall onto my computer but, instead, pool around my neck for easy access.

He added, "Oh wait, almost forgot. The doggie cone has to first be removed from the dog or it won't fit right."

So I suppose you can still binge even when your hands are busy, but your odds are definitely lower. Unless, of course, you have inventive friends like mine. Or you're eating something other than real food. Those imaginary cookies don't require much handling, and they don't drop crumbs on your computer keyboard.

GET A NEW BODITUDE

Questions for Personal Reflection or Group Discussion

- Take an inventory of the majority of foods you eat in any given day. Could they be found growing in a field or produced on a farm? Or are they closer to "foodlike substances," such as chicken fingers?

- When nibbles are prompted by emotions, boredom, or stress, trying to ignore them can be a good strategy. But how often are the food cravings you're trying to ignore inspired by actual hunger? How can you tell the difference?

- How many of your meals or snacks do you wolf down on the go? How often do you eat a meal when you're stressed?

- What do you think of the idea of taking five or ten minutes before a meal to

relax, regroup, count your blessings, or
release the troubles of your day to God?

16
What Happens When Getting What You Want Isn't All It's Cracked Up to Be?

MAKING PEACE WITH SUCCESS

In the months I've been working on this book, I've let a lot of people know I'm in the process of interviewing women who have interesting insights about body image. One evening I received an e-mail from a woman in New York. Her note began with the words, "I received your query from my roommate who works in media . . ."

Heather Waghelstein did, indeed, have a story to tell. My interest was piqued right from the start. She wrote, "When I was eight, my parents took my sister and me shopping for school clothes. My sister had no trouble fitting into the smallest size Jordache jeans, while I sweated and panted with the largest size. I walked out of the mall without new jeans, but carrying a Whopper instead. That was the moment I learned to hate my body — but that feeding it made me feel better." I was even more intrigued when she added this:

My weight fluctuated throughout high school. On my thirtieth birthday I weighed 230 pounds. I started exercising, and by thirty-three I weighed 165 but had mounds of excess skin. I also had jowls, no chin, and thinning hair. On April 15, 2005, I applied to be a guest on the TV reality show *Extreme Makeover* and was accepted. Five months later I was revealed to my family and friends as a size 6, with perfect teeth, a flat stomach, and a smooth jawline. But I still did not feel truly pretty.[1]

A few days later I had Heather on the phone. Almost immediately after exchanging greetings and a few pleasantries, I cut to the chase. "Girlfriend! You were on *Extreme Makeover*! You got the chance to live every woman's dream! Talk to me!"

Heather agreed it was the adventure of a lifetime and that it was truly an "extreme" makeover. In the nearly three months she spent being prepped and filmed for the show, she got the ultimate remodeling. Forget the honey-do list we optimistic women hand the reluctant men in our lives! Heather's Hollywood-do list was embraced enthusiastically by producers, surgeons, and manicurists alike. And by the time her Cinderella adventure came to a close, Heather was not only thirty pounds slimmer, she'd also been remodeled in every other way imaginable. Here's the list of everything that was done:

- hair transplants
- custom hairpieces to make her hair fuller still
- minifacelift
- chin implant
- breast reconstruction
- tummy tuck and back tuck
- liposuction
- new makeup and makeup consultation
- fashion consultation and really cool new clothes
- weight-loss mentoring from diet guru Michael Thurmond
- personal training and workouts four times a week

As she read me the list, I became more convinced than ever that Heather, indeed, had experienced the dream of almost every woman on the planet. I asked her how that felt.

"Out of one hundred thousand applicants,

only one hundred people got to be on the show, and I was one of them," she told me. "So it really was a dream come true. In fact, I remember thinking, *This is it! This is going to solve all of my problems! Everything that has ever bothered me in my entire life is going to be fixed!*"

After the show, before the new-and-improved Heather headed home, the producer asked her how she felt. Heather remembers saying, "Oh, I'm pretty!" Which she definitely was. She was also thrilled and grateful for everything the show had done for her. But there must have been something else that was revealed in her voice, because the producer continued to probe.

"You're usually more thoughtful than that," he said.

Heather hesitated before answering. "It's just the package that looks prettier," she finally said. "But inside I'm still me, and that's the problem."[2]

PERFECT LOOKS, PERFECT LIFE?

It's easy to fall into the trap of believing that if we could just flaunt the right body everything else would fall magically into place. That if our outsides were prettier, our insides would feel healthier. That if we could upgrade our styles, we could begin to accept ourselves. But if this is what we're expecting, we might also discover that success and disillusionment come knockin' hand in hand.

Over the course of a year, a friend of mine lost 120 pounds on a medically supervised liquid fast. In relatively short order, she went from wearing a size 22 to looking like a cover girl. This California blonde had always had a peaches-and-cream complexion and haunting eyes and stunning features, and after losing all that weight, she looked like a model. She says, "I was shocked that, in many ways, my life felt the same. On the surface, everything had changed dramatically, but underneath I still felt lonely and wounded."

This isn't to say that there aren't times when we change something about our bodies or our styles and, as a result, get a new lease on life. I still laugh every time I remember my ten-year-old daughter, who'd grown tired of accompanying her Aunt Michelle and me on a makeup shopping spree. She asked us, as she rolled her eyes, "Why are we even doing this?" To which my sister replied with only partially mock earnestness, "Because, Kaitlyn, the right shade of lipstick can change your entire life."

I can't believe I'm admitting this — again! — but about twelve years ago I had this . . . um . . . tummy tuck. I had just lost sixty pounds and, while my extra padding was gone, the ol' abdomen pouch where I'd once kept all that padding was never going to be the same. So I decided to have a pouchectomy. As I was leaving the doctor's office after a follow-up visit, I thanked him. He said lightly, "Oh, you're welcome," then went on to talk about something else, and I could tell he hadn't really heard me.

I watched his eyes until he looked at me, then held his gaze and said again, more deliberately this time, "Thank you. You have no idea what it's like to be given a second chance like this. Just to be normal again. You have no idea what this means to me. Really. Thank. You."

So sometimes we really can change our bodies or our styles and feel better about ourselves and even life in general. A big external change can have a big impact on us internally. But sometimes the way we feel inside is deep rooted and stubborn. No shade of lipstick will cover it. Losing weight won't shed it. And not even a plastic surgeon's scalpel can cut it away.

"Deep, deep down I know I don't feel as worthy as I should." In the months following her stint on *Extreme Makeover,* Heather thought she was starting a brand-new season, but in many ways her life had returned to its regular programming.

She told me, "I went through this wild phase, going out a lot, trying out my new looks, seeing how many drinks I could get bought for me. I had a couple of casual encounters with men, but it wasn't very fulfilling. And what I discovered is that I was continuing to put myself in the same situations I'd been putting myself in before the makeover, like having casual encounters with men I didn't really care about just to feel loved."

Heather's outward improvements even intensified some of her greatest fears. She explained, "My greatest fear is that I'll be rejected because I'm not willing to sleep with someone. Relationships are always scary for me, and all the increased attention can just make it worse."

Finally, she began to realize that, while success was nice, it didn't pack the same intoxicating punch as the *pursuit* of success. As she explained, "It dawned on me I'd become addicted to dieting. It's a rush see-

241

ing the scale drop another two pounds, or getting into a smaller dress size, or even zipping up your skinny jeans for the first time in months. We chronic dieters love the focus and thrill we get from losing weight, and the only way to keep experiencing these things is to keep losing weight, and the only way to keep losing weight — once you've reached your goal — is to gain it back again."[3]

Heather returned to her job as a recovery-room nurse, working nights. She stopped working out. She started eating cookies at night. She hated the hairpieces so she took them off. Within six months she'd gained twenty pounds. Eventually she would put on more than forty.

Heather's extreme makeover was beginning to come apart at the seams.

CAN WE HANDLE THE RESPONSIBILITY OF SUCCESS?

Success is like a roof. No matter how functional and even beautiful it is, if the architecture of the house beneath it is shaky or compromised, it's going to collapse.

You and I have emotional architecture that either supports the successes we experience or allows those successes to sag and eventually come crashing down around us. Is your emotional architecture sound enough to withstand the weight of success? If we have unrealistic expectations about what losing weight can and cannot do for us . . . if we don't love ourselves to begin with . . . if we are too afraid of rejection to say no to unwanted advances . . . or if we're far more intrigued by the thrill of chasing a goal than by the daily work of maintaining it, we may not yet have the emotional structure in place to hang on to our success.

Heather says she wanted to be a contestant on *Extreme Makeover* to make the way she looked outside match who she thought she was inside. What she didn't realize was that, in many ways, she had already seen to it that her outside and inside matched. Before the makeover, she didn't like the outer Heather, but she didn't love the inner Heather either. After the makeover, she loved the outer Heather but still didn't love the inner Heather. Without realizing it, she had created tension between the crowning glory of her outward success and the inability of her emotions to support that success.

Heather's doing a lot of shoring up, though. Her witty blog — www.fatpantskinny jeans.blogspot.com — chronicles much of her journey. She says it's her way of admitting to herself that she messed up and forgot that loving your body comes from within.

She says she thinks it's best if you can learn to appreciate things about the person you are and the body you have before you go about trying to change everything. She says that even after the makeover, she still saw herself as the fat girl. But as time goes on, she's realizing that she's not.

She admits that deep down she probably doesn't feel as worthy as she should, although she's getting better about this. She went on a date recently with a guy who was all over her. She said, "In the past I probably would have tolerated his hands all over me just because I wanted to be loved. Instead, I walked out. And before I did, I looked at him and said, 'What, are you in high school?'"

She also realized that she's a food addict. She says certain foods, like dairy and chocolate, are to her like whisky is to an alcoholic. She told me, "Today I opened the freezer. My new roommate has chocolate bars in there. I know if I have one, I'll eat them all. It's not even about willpower. I think it's chemical. I can eat carob and stop, but not chocolate. I also see now that, for me, dairy consumption coats me in a layer of fat. I cannot control myself. So last April I became vegan in order to control my food addictions. I eat six times a day, no big meals, all vegan, mostly raw, and only fruit in the morning. I can still have fake cheese and fake meat, which I love, and carob to satisfy my inner chocoholic. This is what works for me."

Finally, she says she's learning the importance of routine. When she returned home from the makeover, she found herself going out a lot more, eating more, drinking more. She says she got out of the routine that had been working for her. Now she tries to be consistent. Not obsessive, just consistent. "If you have a goal, then when you reach that goal you stop doing what you did to get there. Which is why I'm trying to think of this as a long-term thing without a goal or stopping point at the end. Just keep eating well. Eat when I'm hungry. Stop when I'm full. Go running every day with my dog. Just do these things forever and that's all I need to do."

When Heather walked off the set of *Extreme Makeover,* she weighed 136 pounds. These days she fluctuates between 150 and 180. Back in her twenties, she fluctuated between 190 and 230 pounds. She says she's still a yo-yo dieter, but now at least she's yo-yoing in a different range.

I asked if she'd do it all again.

"In a heartbeat. I would do it over and over. I would do it myself if I could afford it. I love what was done. I love that my stomach is flat. Even when I'm bigger — at one-eighty — I love that I'm normal. Curvy, but normal. Can I get back to one hundred thirty-six pounds? I doubt it. Besides, I don't think that's a practical weight for me. I was barely eating in Makeover Land. I don't want to stay at one hundred eighty either, but I like myself. Even with the fluctuations in my weight. I love my body now. I want to take care of it because it's the only one I have."[4]

GET A NEW BODITUDE

Questions for Personal Reflection or Group Discussion
- If you could achieve a dramatic change in the way you look, what do you think that would do for you internally? Do you think an outward change would affect your opinion of yourself?

- Is there any work you need to do now on your emotions so you will be able to hang onto success when it comes? If so, how can you get started on doing that work?

- Have you ever succeeded in changing the way you look only to be disappointed that things you thought would accompany your new body — like relationships, happiness, self-acceptance — didn't happen?

- What is the routine you need to follow in order to have success with your body goals?

17

ONCE UPON
A BRAND-NEW TIME . . .

MAKING PEACE WITH YOUR STORY

You want to know the recipe for a great family road trip? Here it is:

- Take a handful of kids and one or two well-intentioned adults.
- Pack them into a car the size of your average coat closet.
- Jostle, mix, and toss for five to ten days.
- Add PMS, pent-up testosterone, fast-food wrappers, engine trouble, and No Vacancy signs viewed through blood-shot eyes at midnight.
- Marinate in laughter.
- Season stories with a pinch of exaggeration, and enjoy.

Don't you love the stories — from road trips, holidays, and just plain ol' living — that families end up telling and retelling for years to come? Some of these stories are serious, others poignant, and many are hilarious and even inspiring. Then there are stories that get so famous from all the retelling that they become legends in their own right.

Just this morning I was rushing to make school lunches for my daughter Kacie and nephews Hunter and Isaac. Running out of time, I gave them money for the cafeteria instead. As I was doling out the third fiver, I said, "Sheesh, do I look like an ATM to you?" To which Isaac quipped, "Do I look like a fanny pack to you?" and the four of us busted up laughing.

Why did we laugh so heartily at what an uninitiated onlooker would consider inane? That, my friend, is the power of the inside joke. Only Kacie, Isaac, Hunter, their brother Connor, and I know the unabridged story behind the hilarious nine-word punch line Isaac used to reduce us to weak-kneed, teary-eyed belly laughter. No small achievement at 6:20 in the morning, I might add.

But that's the point. Stories, if they're told often enough, become more than stories. They become emotional quick links that transport us into whatever state of mind or spirit we were in back when the story was a brand-new experience.

That is the power — and, of course, the danger — of our stories.

The Stories That Created You

Fill in the blank: "Today, I have the relationship I have with my body because _____."

There is a story, or more likely a series of stories, that come together to form what you think about yourself, your body, and your life. The best stories are told and retold. They capture the imagination of listeners. Friends ask: "And then what happened?"

Stories also play a central role in getting to know someone, and in inviting another person to get to know you. A new friend will ask: "Tell me about yourself!" or "So! How did you two meet?"

Years pass, and the answers take on a repetitive sameness. They are not lifeless, because rarely does a good story become lifeless. But the words can be repeated verbatim, as if by spinning the same phrases over and over, they've been embroidered into the fabric of your identity.

This is all well and good if the story's punch line evokes laughter and delight, or delivers a happy ending after a few suspenseful subplots. If the story leaves listeners (as well as the teller) feeling inspired and grateful, the story is cherished.

But some stories are dark or damaging. And even though we may not tell such stories in public, we continue to repeat those stories to ourselves. These are the stories we tell ourselves about our relationships with food, exercise, self-esteem, and more. These stories explain what lies behind our struggles:

- "Why do I hate my body?"
- "Why do I feel so unworthy?"
- "What happened to convince me that I'm not as pretty as I should be?"
- "Why do I feel so broken inside?"
- "Why do I hate exercise?"
- "When did I make food my best friend?"

A number of women have told their dark stories throughout this book. Jeacline admitted that she started dieting at age seven and always thought she needed to be thinner to be perfect. My story is that I'm afraid of painful emotions and will do anything — including eat myself into a carb coma — to avoid them. Karen Kartes used exercise to keep her body from developing the womanly curves that were characteristic of other women in her family. When our princess in chapter 12 felt unloved, food salved her pain, and the weight she gained helped solve the mystery of rejection in her marriage.

Laura Fenamore, who happens to be a Body Image Mastery mentor, explains: "We each have a story about why our body is the way it is. Many times other people helped create this story. Some stories are kinder than others. But they shape our body image as we grow up. . . . So how do we know when a story is healthy or not? How do we know if a story is trapping us? That takes being really honest with yourself and admitting whether your story empowers you to get the results you desire, or if it empowers you to justify the results you have."

Laura gives several examples of unhealthy stories that not only describe yesterday's events, but determine today's choices:

"I've never had control over what happens to me or in my life. The only control I have is whether I eat and what I eat."

"My home was a wreck. There was always fighting. Food was my only solace. It still is my safety net and friend."

"In gym class, I was always made fun of for being clumsy. It was painful always being the last kid picked for a team. Physical activities always make me feel inadequate or incompetent."

"I'm proud of the fact that I have no boundaries around food. I eat whatever I want, when I want. Those people who diet and worry about what they eat are kidding themselves."

"Being heavy my whole life prevented me from [developing] hand-eye coordination and balance. It's impossible for me to try to be active now."[1]

STORIES THAT DELIVER INSIGHT

There's a book I love by Jon Franklin called *Writing for Story.* In it he talks about techniques and principles of writing, and discusses something he calls "the point of insight." Throughout most of a story, the main character bumbles along, trying to solve her problem while encountering obstacle after obstacle. Somewhere near the end of the story, she has a flash of insight and realizes what she must do to solve her problem. Then she solves her problem and the story ends.

Our heroine will struggle along in one direction — perhaps for years — until something shifts. Suddenly she's headed in a new direction, toward a solution and the happy ending she craves. I'm not saying her problem is suddenly solved, or even that it will be solved in short order. Her journey toward a solution will almost always take lots of effort and time — weeks or months or even years. But she's on the right path now, and making progress every day.

This is the point of insight. It's the moment when our friend Jeacline, stricken with colon cancer, chose to jettison dissatisfaction and ungratefulness and instead decided to be happy and grateful for her body and her life.

The point of insight for Danielle came when she started appreciating the body she has, making a commitment to wear beautiful, right-fitting clothing regardless of the number on her scale.

In the movie *Baby Boom,* this is the moment Manhattan executive-turned-rural-single-mom J. C. Wiatt realized that, instead of giving in to feeling frumpy, depressed, and aimless in her farmhouse, she could . . . make applesauce! By starting a business and embracing (and eventually loving) her new life, J. C. (Diane Keaton) found herself well on the road to happiness, success, and true love.

Some points of insight we've heard about in this book were my daughter Kaitlyn's looking in the mirror and speaking words of grace and truth over her body, the moment Mary began loving her polio-stricken body through poetry, the moment Karen Kartes heard God whispering to her through her anorexia-induced despair and realized she was loved and accepted for who she is.

It's the moment Cinderella realizes that, if she's ever going to have the life she wants, she'll have to leave the cage of roles and expectations that her stepfamily built for her, step up to the glass slipper, and put it on.

Sometimes — in movies and in real life too — we come to a crossroads. We can continue on the path we've been traveling, or we can strike off in an entirely new direction. The choice is ours.

A BLAST AWAY FROM THE PAST

One of the perks of being self-employed and working as a writer is that I often get to speak to groups. I've spoken at community fund-raisers, church services, and women's retreats. Once I spoke at a Valentine's Day event where they served wine and one guy got tipsy and kept interrupting my speech. I did a book signing at Borders while wearing pajamas. My daughters say I even speak in my sleep. (Once, while asleep, I announced the formula for capturing space aliens.)

I also speak at writers' workshops, and when I do, pretty much anything can happen. The last time I did a workshop for writers, I wore my belly-dancing skirt, staged a mock fight, and released my hyper Boston terrier unannounced into the room. I've asked writers to create narrative from odd and untested perspectives, say from the viewpoint of a coffee pot. (I'll never look at a seemingly innocent cup of coffee in the same light again.)

There's one writing exercise I ask my writers to do that I think will benefit you and me. I call it "Honey, Oprah's hologram just showed up in the video-tube." Imagine this. It's five years from now, and Oprah calls and invites you to be a guest on her show. She says America is literally salivating to hear what you have to say.

Once you're there, in front of an attentive studio audience and with cameras rolling, Oprah looks at you and says earnestly, "For years you struggled to change your body, love yourself, and transform your life. You tried fad diets. You experienced temporary success and devastating setbacks. You felt trapped and wondered if you would ever find a way to make peace with the things that were making you dissatisfied with yourself."

(Women in the studio audience and in living rooms across America are listening, mesmerized, while wiping tears from their eyes.)

Oprah leans close and asks, "So, how did you do it? How did you get from where you were — let's say, five years ago — to where you are today? What was the turning point? How did you finally — finally! — find a way to make peace with food, make peace with your body, and perhaps most important of all, make peace with your emotions about your body? Tell us your story!"

That's my question for you, and it makes an excellent writing exercise. Five years from now, what will your story be? I imagine it will begin with the part of the story you would tell me today if I asked why your body is the way it is, or why sometimes you feel powerless to change your life. Perhaps you would say . . .

"I always felt unloved and vulnerable and inadequate . . ."

"I had always turned to food when . . ."

"I couldn't seem to shake the feeling that I didn't deserve love or happiness . . ."

"I used food to manage my emotions and solve my dilemmas . . ."

"During my childhood I never felt good enough, then when I got to college . . .

"I never had a weight problem until my divorce, but then my life was turned upside down, and I began . . ."

Go ahead. Tell me this part of your story.

Right here:

STANDING AT THE CROSSROADS

Now it gets fun and interesting. Because today, right now, you have arrived at the crossroads. Today is where you get to decide to take a different path. Today is where your story veers in a new direction and you can decide to stop letting yesterday's hurts, limitations, and obstacles determine what happens tomorrow, and the next day, and the days and months and years after that.

What is your turning point? Pretend you are looking back on your life from five years into the future, and tell me about your point of insight. What realization have you come to? Perhaps you'll write:

"One morning I woke up and realized . . ."

"I still remember the day . . ."

"One day my husband said to me . . ."

"It wasn't a single moment, but a series of successes that made me realize . . ."

"It was when the doctor said to me . . ."

"I got sick and tired of hating myself and made a decision to . . ."

And of course my personal favorite: "I read this book by Karen Linamen that changed my life forever . . ."

But don't let me put words in your mouth. Below, tell me about the crossroads you have reached, and describe the insight or event that is going to cause you to take the road untraveled.

A NEW STORY

Now here's where you get to be *really* creative, because I want you to tell me the new things you did and experienced as a result of taking that new path. I realize you haven't done these things yet. That's okay. Picture them and then describe them. If we were in one of my writing workshops, I'd tell you this is where you get to practice your fiction-writing skills. In fact, let your imagination run wild, and imagine all sorts of new choices and new thoughts and wonderful new experiences — then write about them as if they have already come to pass.

Whatever you come up with will be great. Even if it feels like wishful thinking, or seems highly unlikely. What matters is that you're giving your brain permission to believe there's a new, healthy direction to take from where you are today, a turn that will get you to where you want to be. You're creating a path, and as you look into your own future, your brain knows there *is* a better path to take. Your spirit and your emotions know it too. And once you've been there in your imagination, you can find your way there again, this time for real.

Need a few ideas?

"The first thing I did was join a gym. I started out by standing on a treadmill like that crazy Linamen chick suggested — and you know what? It made a difference! I began loving the way I felt about my body. Before long I upgraded all my lingerie. I wasn't at my perfect weight, but I didn't care. I wanted to celebrate the way I was feeling about myself. Six months later I was asked to teach an exercise class at church . . ."

"I started standing naked in front of a mirror and speaking truth about my body . . ."

"I took a nutrition class . . ."

"I found a wonderful counselor who helped me . . ."

"I wrote an article about my journey, and it was published in a national women's magazine . . ."

". . . which is about the time I wrote a letter to my family releasing them from . . ."

"I took the affirmation statements I'd written for myself, reproduced them on three-by-five cards, and started selling them online. Now I not only feel beautiful and confident about my body, but I've just made my first million . . ."

". . . which is when Larry King asked me about . . ."

"I taped pictures of plus-size models all over my bathroom mirror to remind myself that you don't have to look like Barbie to be beautiful."

". . . about that time, my girlfriends and I painted our bodies and ran naked through a moonlit forest . . ."

"Six months after I stopped using my weight to push men away and welcomed the thought that I deserved love, I met this great guy who loves me for me. We're married now and have two beautiful children."

"I figured the best way to grasp my true purpose and design was to get to know the One who made me, so I decided to . . ."

"I stopped thinking of myself as damaged goods and started picturing myself as whole, healthy, and happy . . ."

"I followed Mary's example and starting writing poetry in which I envisioned . . ."

". . . now roughly nine million people follow me on Twitter . . ."

"I knew I had finally made peace with the things that were making me feel bad about my body and myself when . . ."

". . . and now they are making this documentary about my life, which will be aired in eleven-minute segments on YouTube . . ."

Get crazy. Dream big. Five years from now, what would you love to be telling Oprah about your new story as it's going to unfold starting today? Jot it down here:

My Story

I've asked you to rewrite the ending to the story you've been telling yourself. So I owe it to you — and to myself — to do the same. I'm going to write my own story, including old insights from the past, newly acquired insights from this book, and my vision for my future. It will be a blend of fact and fiction, to be sure. (When I get to the part where I'm writing about my vision for my future, I'll indent the text so things won't get confusing. But if you ask me, the fiction part may be the most important of all.)

Here goes: I'm not a girl who is brave in the face of conflict. I love peace and harmony. I love encouragement and kind words. Oh, and I don't like pain. At some point in my twenties, when facing pain I didn't know how to handle, I turned to food. I continued turning to food to avoid pain, which, of course, created new pain. And that pain sent me foraging for more food, which created more pain. Pretty soon I began to believe the lie that the only way to stay safe — particularly from relationship stress or pain — was to stay fat, which of course didn't keep me safe at all. Although sometimes it gave me the illusion of being safer, but only because being heavy created its own body of pain that was so large it eclipsed all the other sources of pain in my life.

Having struggled with this for twenty years, one day I decided to write a book and call it *A Waist Is a Terrible Thing to Mind* (which, as we know, it certainly is!). And, of course, when I started writing this book, I envisioned it as a great way to lose a hundred pounds and show up all toned and svelte on the cover of *Woman's Day* or maybe even *Redbook.* Which was ridiculous because the book I was writing wasn't supposed to be about losing weight.

Instead, the book was about making peace with the things that make women — me included — feel bad about their bodies. I figured I'd learn a lot along the way. But even I was surprised by the unexpected things I learned. Here's the short list of insights I've gained from this project:

I loved learning about Joe Ramirez's three-hour rule, which says I need to think about how much movement I'll be doing in the next three hours and eat carbs accordingly. Another great insight from Joe is that people who keep food logs lose twice the weight as people who don't. I'm also thrilled that Joe helped me — finally! — understand how my metabolism really works, and that there are things I can do to speed it up. From the first day I contacted him, Joe gave me hope and optimism, which was priceless.

I was moved by the comments I read on www.experienceproject.com, posted by women expressing their feelings about their bodies. I related more than I thought I would to their angst.

Jenny Craig's insights about the link between negative self-talk and stress and weight loss were fascinating. I've always been convinced that what we say to ourselves about ourselves matters, and her words left me more convinced than ever that my negative self-talk was hurting me in ways I hadn't realized. I was also surprised by some of my long-ago memories that were evoked as I wrote on this topic, memories of old criticisms I thought I'd laid to rest.

As I wrote about making peace with our emotions . . . wow! There was a lot of personal discovery that took place as I realized for the first time how hard I try to avoid, not just actual hurt, but even *potential* hurt. I also realized how I'd been using my body to buffer that pain, and I even wrote a letter to my body, saying, "Thank you for stepping up to the plate and shouldering the insane responsibility I've asked you to carry." I released my body from that burden in the future, promising to find healthy ways to cope with real and potential hurt.

But I think the stories from the women who contacted me impacted me more than anything else. Heather's insights really struck me, and a light went on when she talked about regaining weight being the only way to later experience the thrill of coming back down the scale. Karen Kartes's story left me struggling — in a good way! — to think about my own narrow definition of beauty. Jill's angst — and solution — when her husband said her weight was driving him to an affair impacted me hugely. I felt personally encouraged when I read about Andrea's decision to love and respect her curvy body, as well as Danielle's insights about dressing well at any size. And I was absolutely inspired when my mom embraced weight training for the first time in her life.

Laura's insights into the power of our stories felt like strong hands merging with mine to shape the clay of my long-held convictions on this matter and, in fact, gave me the strength to revisit my own story.

Kaitlyn's story reminded me that there are magical things taking place all around us — sometimes under our own roofs — and that sometimes we are blessed enough to discover them.

Finally, Jeacline's story had such a personal impact that I cried, then wrote her a letter promising that I would, indeed, listen to what she was telling me and stop the mental merry-go-round of doubts and insecurities that I'd been spinning.

I know I'm at a crossroads. I can continue on my old path or take a new one, and I have decided to change my story. So here goes:

In the five years since I finished this book, I decided to stop letting yesterday's hurts, experiences, limitations, and perspectives determine what happens for me tomorrow, and the next day, and the days and months and years after that.

I started jogging again (I'd started while writing this book but had been slacking off). I stopped feeling sorry for myself. I began rewarding my body with healthy food instead of junk food. I asked God to help me understand more of his amazing design for who he created me to be. I stopped revisiting my old story, going back to the hurts and the pity parties. Sometimes I've wondered if emotional pain and even critical self-talk are like the sore spots we get in our mouths. There is some comfort to be found in poking at that spot with our tongues. But for the first time in a long time, I decided to do everything in my power (asking God to help me) to stop poking around the sore spots and let them finally heal.

Oh, and get this! Shortly after this book became a *New York Times* bestseller, I was checking out of a ritzy hotel in Chicago (I'd flown into town so I could appear on *Oprah.* I KNOW! Wild, huh?) when I spotted a familiar face from my past! It was a dear friend I hadn't seen in years. Linda was in Chicago on business and about to meet several colleagues for lunch. Since my plane didn't leave until that evening, I joined them. Turns out one of the guys in the group and I had a lot in common. No, he doesn't belly dance, but he does own a pirate costume, and while he's never been felled by a chairlift, he told me that when he was a baby, he tumbled out of his stroller once, which is close enough for me. We're madly in love and are planning a chocolate-themed wedding in the fall.

Sometimes I still eat for comfort or to avoid painful emotions. But it's not very often now, and, when it happens, I see it as the glitch it is, forgive myself, and move on. I've found a weight that's healthy for me and have managed to stay within about twelve pounds of that weight. But whether I'm at the top end of my range or the bottom, I'm okay. I'm thankful for the beautiful body given to me by my Creator, and, most important, I'm thrilled that he loves and values me, inside and out, no matter what I weigh.

Don't you love stories in which some unexpected discovery changes the course of everything? Those stories don't just happen on the big screen, or in fairy tales, or even in books like this one. They happen in real life too. Furthermore, they can happen in *your* life.

What are we waiting for, you and I? Our stories — at least our stories about our relationships with our bodies — are being written even as we speak. And here's the best news of all: we're the ones holding the ballpoint pen!

GET A NEW BODITUDE

Questions for Personal Reflection or Group Discussion
- Have you held on to a story that is keeping you from making the changes you long to make in your life? If so, what is the story? What keeps you hanging on to the old story?

- If you could embrace a new story, what would it be?

- Are there stories and insights in this book that have given you some life-changing ideas? Name three of them.

- How would you like the next five years of your life to unfold? Are you willing to write down your dreams and goals with confident expectation, as if they had already occurred?

- What obstacles can you think of that could keep your life from unfolding in the way you've just described? Can you edit these obstacles out of your story? If not, can you write in a solution to each one? Now is the time to get started.

NOTES

Chapter 3

1. See Karen Scalf Linamen, *Only Nuns Change Habits Overnight* (Colorado Springs, CO: WaterBrook, 2008).
2. Jack Hollis, quoted in Bonnie Schiedel, "Why Keeping a Food Journal Will Help You Lose Weight," *Best Health Magazine,* January/February 2009, www.besthealth mag.ca/eat-well/diet/why-keeping-a-food-journal-will-help-you-lose-weight.
3. See www.todaysdietandnutrition.com/oct06health.shtml?action=results&poll_ident=8.

Chapter 4

1. Quotes obtained during a telephone interview with Jenny Craig, September 22, 2009. Used by permission.
2. Robert Moss, "Thoughts Can Heal Your Body," March 9, 2008, *Parade.com,* www .parade.com/articles/editions/2008/

edition_03-09-2008/2Thoughts_Can_Heal.

3. Maxwell Maltz, *Psycho-Cybernetics* (Englewood Cliffs, NJ: Pocket Books, 1960), 2.

Chapter 7

1. For more information about our writers' group, go to www.meetup.com/occwriters.

Chapter 9

1. Dr. Roger Gould, "Article 2: Food Addiction and How It Starts," www.shrinkyourself.com/ee_101_join.asp.

2. See www.addictionsandrecovery.org/recovery-skills.htm.

3. Author's paraphrase of the famous biblical story. To read the entire account, see Matthew 14:22–33.

Chapter 10

1. Karen Kartes's story was obtained in a telephone interview with the author, June 30, 2009. Used by permission.

Chapter 12

1. Anna Stookey's comments are taken from her blog, www.bodyreunion.blogspot.com. Used by permission.

Chapter 13

1. "Maintaining Aerobic Fitness Could Delay Biological Aging By Up to 12 Years, Study Shows," *Science Daily,* April 10, 2008, www.sciencedaily.com/releases/2008/04/080409205827.htm.

2. Anne Underwood, "Check Out Grandma's Biceps!: New research shows that exercise can help reverse the aging process at the cellular level. Strength training for the senior set," *Newsweek,* May 22, 2007, www.newsweek.com/id/34489.

3. You can learn more about the work of Janine Hightower at www.bostonhomebodies.com.

4. Mary McManus's story was obtained in an interview with the author on August 3, 2009. Used by permission. You can learn more about Mary and her books of poetry at www.newworldgreetings.com.

5. Jeacline's story is taken from e-mail correspondence with the author and is used by permission. You can find her blog at www.cancerwarrior.wordpress.com, and you can e-mail her at Jeacline@1SmartHealthCoach.com.

Chapter 14

1. See www.getromantic.com/passion/spice_up_sex/mistakes_women_make.html.

2. Yvonne Fulbright, "12 Things You Should Never Do When It Comes to Sex," *FoxNews.com,* July 16, 2009, www.fox news.com/story/0,2933,533260,00.html ?sPage=fnc/health/men.

Chapter 15
1. You can read more about Diana Walker's work, and benefit from her advice, at www .thecravingscoach.com.
2. See http://thecravingscoach.com/blog/ relaxation-meditation-helps-curb-cravings.

Chapter 16
1. Heather Waghelstein e-mail to the author, June 23, 2009. Used by permission.
2. Heather Waghelstein, in a telephone interview with the author on September 3, 2009. Used by permission.
3. Waghelstein, telephone interview.
4. Waghelstein, telephone interview.

Chapter 17
1. Laura Fenamore's comments were obtained from correspondence with the author, June 23, 2009. Used by permission. You can read more about Laura's work and sign up for her free newsletter at www.onepinky.com.